Younger You

Younger Me

Barbara A. Hoffman

*How to Feel & Look Young
Into Your 90's and Beyond!*

Younger You
Younger Me

By Barbara A. Hoffman

Disclaimer:
This book is intended as a reference volume only, not as a medical manual. The information given here is designed to help you make informed decisions about your health. The dietary programs in this book are not intended as a substitute for any dietary regimen that may have been prescribed by your doctor. If you have a medical condition you should discuss all new dietary programs with your doctor before beginning.

First Edition: February 2013. Printed in the USA.
International Standard Book number:

Trademarks
All terms mentioned in this book that are known to be trademarks or service marks have been appropriately capitalized. Trademarks belong to the appropriate companies.

About The Author

Barbara A. Hoffman

Barbara Hoffman is a Naturopath, medical researcher & journalist, women's health advocate and natural hormone and weight consultant.

For 10 years she produced a cable network television program which focused on health and wellness. Her passion to teach fuels her mission to empower women to make better educated, informed choices about their health.

Barbara has been in the medical field for over thirty years and worked in the field of women's health since 1980. For the past twenty years she has been researching weight loss, the benefits of natural progesterone and writing about alternatives to synthetic hormones. Her focus continues to be natural hormones but she has a passion for women & men who are lugging around 20 – 40 extra pounds and who tell her they just "feel old". Her message is: There is HOPE and it's not difficult to regain your youthful vigor!

Barbara currently resides in Orange County, California. She has been happily married for 26 years and has one son.

Dedication

- I dedicate this book to all of you who find life to be a grand, God-given adventure. You are committed to be your best "you" and you will inspire others. On we go to longevity and vitality into our 90's and beyond. We need to live a long & healthy, energetic life because that is God's plan for us.

- My Lord & God from whom all Blessings Flow.
  As for me, & my house (and office), we will always serve You.

- I also salute 2 people who keep me always on my toes to be a Younger Barbara:

  Jessica Prussa – The best office "production manager" ever.
  Nicole Pillsbury – My Assistant "Extraordinaire" & "stylist" who encourages me daily. She also loves to encourage all of you who call or write. What a Beautiful Heart.

- Finally, to David & Drew; God's gifts to me. You keep me true of heart and I love you more than words can ever say.

That's all – Go Forth and change your world!

Love,
Barbara
June 2013

The Secret To The Younger YOU

Hello Friends:

Have you decided that you want to look younger or feel younger? Have you thought about it for many years but don't know where to start?

Well I want to tell you that those women you see who are walking by, looking younger than you (although you suspect they are older than you) they are working at it.

And you can, too. I know that I am not getting younger but I feel so young and vibrant because of simple steps that I take and you can too. It's never too late to start.

You don't have to do everything right away. Start with small steps and move forward. I'll be with you all the way.

I am going to give you my best tips. It is a fun and satisfying journey.

You can be a younger YOU . . . until the end of your earthly days.

I urge you to look in the mirror. Think back over the last 5 years. Do you feel that you have aged? If so, time to take action. You can turn back the clock.

You can look younger, have younger energy and have a younger attitude.

Your age is just a number. It does not define you. Your spirit is what shows people who you are. I urge you not to worry when you turn that calendar every year on your birthday. Instead, I want you to concentrate on getting younger during that year. That will excite you. It's a challenge. And that's what this book is meant to do. Challenge you to be the younger you.

Have you noticed that even advertisers are now realizing that older people are still appealing? There are more and more pictures of people our age in commercials. The sense of who looks attractive has changed and that's great for Younger you, Younger me.

At any age you can be one of the most beautiful women or most handsome man on earth. Yes, you can ......on into our 50s, 60s, 70s, 80s and 90s. We are going to embrace these years as powerful wonderful fruit-bearing years that we will savor to the fullest.

We are going to leave this earth still having fun, still playing, and still having people attracted to our youthful spirit.

Yes we are. Let's get started.

Don't settle for feeling or looking older than your years.

It's all here . . . what you need to know to be a Younger You.

Younger You
Younger Me

Table of Contents

Part I – Living Your Life As The Younger You

Part II – Looking Like The Younger You

Dear Reader:
This book is divided into categories
for your reading convenience.

What is you main concern?
Flip to the pertinent chapter for the keys to
erasing years off your body and mind.

Part I

Living Your Life As The
Younger You

Chapter 1

Hormone Balance

I always start here when I talk to you on the phone or in emails. Hormone balance is the key to feeling youthful! If our hormones are out of balance we are not going to feel good and consequently we will not look good either. I am going to show you how to be hormonally balanced at any age. It is not difficult.

I firmly believe that "feeling old" starts when hormones begin to become unbalanced. For women, you can become exhausted, can't sleep, have night sweats, mood swings, aches and pains that you never had before. You feel miserable and therefore you feel old and rundown. For men, the same thing occurs when hormone levels are not balanced. Your body begins to malfunction in big ways or small ways. In men, this is called andro-pause. In women, it's peri-menopause or menopause or, as some women have called it "mean-pause" or "men-pause". Libido and mood truly suffer for both sexes during these times. Without our happy mood and vibrant libido, we feel old.

When we enter menopause, (starting with peri-menopause) or for the men, andro-pause, our age physiologically begins to decline. Lack of hormones accelerates the process. For men andro-pause will start after the age of 40. For women, the symptoms of menopause can begin when they're in their 30's and last for years until you reach the age of 50-51.

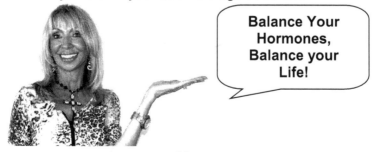

Balance Your Hormones, Balance your Life!

The changes creep up slowly, but sure enough we start to feel we're not the "person we used to be." In other words, an older version of ourselves.

Andro-pause and menopause can lead to osteoporosis, dry skin and hair, increased body fat, and interference with your thyroid hormones. And let's not forget memory loss, which can be quite frightening for us. Here's what you need to know to balance those hormones and get you back to that youthful you.

What are the symptoms of hormone imbalance?
Here they are. Read them, but don't weep. We can fix this problem! (Some of these are exclusive to women.)

1. Hot flashes, flushes, night sweats and/or cold flashes, feeling clammy
2. Irregular heart beat
3. Irritability
4. Mood swings, sudden tears
5. Trouble sleeping through the night
6. Irregular periods; shorter, lighter periods; heavier periods, flooding; shorter cycles, longer cycles
7. Loss of libido
8. Dry vagina
9. Crashing fatigue
10. Anxiety, feeling ill at ease
11. Feelings of dread, apprehension, doom
12. Difficulty concentrating, disorientation, mental confusion
13. Disturbing memory lapses
14. Incontinence, especially upon sneezing, laughing
15. Itchy, crawly skin
16. Aching, sore joints, muscles and tendons
17. Increased tension in muscles
18. Breast tenderness
19. Headache change: increase or decrease
20. Gastrointestinal distress, indigestion, flatulence, nausea
21. Sudden bouts of bloat
22. Depression
23. Exacerbation of existing conditions

24. Increase in allergies
25. Weight gain
26. Hair loss/thinning, head, pubic, or whole body; increased facial hair
27. Dizziness, light-headedness, episodes of loss of balance
28. Changes in body odor
29. Electric shock sensation under the skin and in the head
30. Tingling in the extremities
31. Gum problems, increased bleeding
32. Burning tongue, burning roof of mouth, bad taste in mouth, change in breath odor
33. Osteoporosis (after several years)
34. Changed in fingernails: softer, crack or break easier
35. Tinnitus: ringing in ears, bells, 'whooshing,' buzzing etc.

What Can You Do?

Progesterone can help. I believe God gave us progesterone to keep us balanced and to keep us young. Progesterone is a natural anti-anxiety and stress reliever. It balances cortisol levels, and calms the brain by increasing GABA.

GABA is Gamma-aminobutyric-Acid, an amino acid that is the 2nd most common neurotransmitter in the brain. Without GABA, a person would constantly remain on edge, anxious and not have the ability to relax.

Progesterone also is a vasodilator. It can help lower blood pressure and help protect your heart. Progesterone also can help protect against breast cancer. It can help with your weight by instructing the body to BURN the food that you eat for energy instead of storing it as FAT. It can also help improve serotonin levels and promote better sleep. It restores libido in many people and also protects the thyroid. Progesterone can lower insulin levels and help you have a better lipid profile. Wow! This is the "hormone of youth", in my opinion.

Where Can I Get It?

In the U.S., it is available without a prescription, in other words, over-the-counter. AND, it's not expensive. A jar of USP progesterone can be purchased for under $30.

How do I use progesterone?
Menstruating women: (including Peri-Menopause) Apply
1/4 tsp. twice daily on inner arms, wrists, palms of hands, neck
or inner thighs. Start on the 12th day after first day of
menstrual flow through 26th day. Repeat monthly.
Occasionally rotate areas of application.
Non-menstruating women: Apply 1/4 tsp. twice daily on inner
arms, wrists, palms of hands, neck or inner thighs. Use 25
days per month. Repeat monthly.

Men: Use ¼ tsp. once daily of a 500 mg cream. If using a
1000 mg cream, use 1/8 tsp. once a day. Men do NOT need
time off like women and can take the progesterone without
taking any days off. Occasionally rotate areas of application.
(We will talk more about the men in chapter 13.)

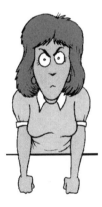

PMS (Pre-menopausal Symptom) makes
women feel cranky and old before their
time. For women, hormone imbalance can
begin in your teens and last for years if not
addressed. This is known as Pre-
menstrual Syndrome (PMS). Studies
indicate that the worse your PMS is when
you are young, the worse your menopause
will be.
PMS is characterized by a set of hormonal
changes that trigger disruptive symptoms
for up to two weeks prior to menstruation.

Causes
PMS seems to be related to fluctuations in estrogen and
progesterone levels in the body, especially a condition termed
Estrogen Dominance.

Women feel "out-of-control", anxious, depressed, can have
uncontrollable crying spells. Other common complaints are
headache and fatigue.
When you are experiencing PMS, it will make you look cranky
& irritable which translates to looking like a "meanie" No! We
want to look calm, peaceful and glowing. It's hard to glow
when you're PMSing.

Progesterone can correct PMS in 1 – 3 cycles. Back to feeling good! Just use from day 12 – 26 of each cycle.

"What about HRT? That's what my doctor gave me."
I say that It's A 'Syn' To Be On Synthetics!

Synthetic hormones have terrible side effects including breast cancer, heart attack, stroke and blood clots. Another significant side effect is weight gain. Yikes! Extra weight makes us look slower, tired, takes the "spring" out of our step. Not to mention the double-chin and muffin top. Some women have gained up to 40 pounds on HRT.

Here are my Top Reasons
To Get Off Synthetic HRT

1. On July 9, 2002, the National Institutes of Health **HALTED** a landmark scientific study of synthetic hormone replacement therapy (Premarin and Provera) because they found that synthetic estrogen / progestin therapy resulted in: <u>**41% increased risk of stroke, 29% increased risk of heart attack, 26% increased risk of breast cancer and a doubled rate of blood clots in the legs and lungs**</u> when compared to women on no hormone therapy.

2. **Premarin is not "natural" to the human body.** It is made from pregnant mare's urine. The generic name for Premarin is conjugated equine estrogen. There are hundreds of different horse estrogen compounds contained in Premarin, which are foreign to the human body. **Also, Premarin contains large amounts of Estrone, which can stimulate breast cells.** In 1995 the American Journal of Obstetrics and Gynecology published a study stating that long-term AND short-term users of Premarin had a **40% risk of acquiring breast cancer.**

3. Feb 13, 2002 - Journal of the American Medical Society - study of HRT in Relation to Breast Cancer. Results showed that longer use of HRT was associated with increased risk of breast cancer. The incidence of **breast cancer was increased by 60% to 85%** in recent long-term users of HRT.

4. The estrogen, "estriol" is completely missing from most forms of conventional HRT. Estriol protects the body from the proliferative effects (causing cells to multiply) estrone and estradiol and is especially protective against breast cancer.

5. Two new studies show **SYNTHETIC HORMONE THERAPY IS LINKED TO BRAIN SHRINKAGE.** The studies show that commonly prescribed forms of postmenopausal hormone therapy may slightly accelerate the loss of brain tissue in women 65 and older beyond what normally occurs with aging.

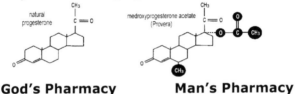

God's Pharmacy   **Man's Pharmacy**

9. A side effect of synthetic hormones is **weight gain**, especially around the middle, hips and thighs (the classic "pear-shaped" weight gain. The average weight gain in women who were placed on synthetic hormones was between 20-30 pounds, sometimes even more!

16

Examples of Artificial / Synthetic Hormones

ESTROGENS: *Premarin, Cenestin, Menest, OrthoEst, EstraTab.*

PROGESTERONES (called progestins): *Provera, Aygestin and DepoProvera and certain birth control pills.*

COMBINATIONS: *EstraTest, Activella, PremPro, PremPhase, CombiPatch, ClimaraPro, FemHRT*, and *110 types of hormonal birth control methods.*

Testosterone: *MethylTestosterone*

When correcting hormonal imbalance, it is common sense to use the exact human hormones(s) that are needed. Drug companies make chemically altered synthetic drugs because this allows them to patent their products which yields protected BIG revenue. Altered chemical structure means VERY different actions in the body.

"Or do you not know that your body is a temple of the Holy Spirit within you, whom you have from God? You are not your own, for you were bought with a price.
So glorify God in your body."
1 Corinthians 6:19-20

Chapter 2

Energy: Essential to Youthfulness

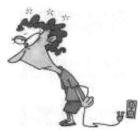

If you are over the age of 45, you may have noticed that you feel tired and drained of energy more frequently. Do you find yourself frequently nodding off in front of the t.v.? Have you heard yourself saying "I don't have the energy I used to"? You think that this could simply be due to the ageing process. However, feeling old and feeling tired do not have to go hand-in-hand. I want you to be *Retired*, NOT *Tired*. Feeling low on energy is not a condition that you should.

Good energy is a sign that our body is running on all cylinders. Low energy can be due to a lack of sleep. You should be getting 7-8 hours of sleep per night. Older adults spend less time in a deep sleep, which is the most restful phase of sleep. (We will discuss insomnia in chapter 14.)

In the meantime, your lack of energy can be a symptoms of a low hormone. That hormone is DHEA and it is my all-time favorite supplement for energy is a hormone,

(DeHydroEpiAndrosterone) DHEA
DHEA is the #1 Supplement recommended by Age-Management Doctors worldwide! It is often referred to as *"The Hormone of Youth"*.

Studies suggest that anyone over the age of 40 should be taking DHEA! Why is that?
DHEA levels peak at the age of 20 for both men and women and can go downhill from there.

Declining DHEA levels are believed to be associated with arthritis, memory loss, heart disease, low libido, belly fat and loss of energy.
DHEA is good for the brain too. Research studies show that DHEA supplementation has an anti-depressant effect. It also protects from cortisol overconcentration.

Is It Safe?
DHEA is all-natural and very safe to use when taken at the normal physiological dose.

"I have noticed that DHEA users have a renewed vigor & energy. They also seem to do better with their chronic health conditions."- *Dr. L. Yu (Orthomolecular Medicine)*

What Can It Do For You?
- Improve Vitality and Energy
- Increases muscle mass, & better muscle tone
- Improves memory & recall
- Helps relieve hot flashes
- Increases testosterone levels
- Increases libido in both sexes
- Aid weight loss; prevent accumulation of belly fat Women who received DHEA lost an average of 10.2% of their visceral fat, while men lost an average of 7.4%. Impressive!
- Enhances the thermogenic process (Food is converted to energy instead of fat)
- Enhances mood, relieves depression
- Supports hormone balance & regulates thyroid gland
- Can reduce insulin, glucose & cholesterol levels
- Has anti-dementia effects
- Counter-balances cortisol
- Skin appears smoother & better hydrated
- Improves energy & adrenal health & increases stamina
- Lowers blood cholesterol levels
- Promotes better sleep
- Decreases the stickiness of platelets, to help prevent heart attacks and strokes

- Support adrenal health
- <u>Longer Life</u>: A 12 year study published in the New England Journal of Medicine in 1986 showed that increases in DHEA levels corresponded with a 36% reduction in mortality rates.
- Can increase bone density to prevent or reduce osteoporosis
- DHEA has also been helpful in the treatment of
  - Alzheimer's
  - Multiple sclerosis
  - Memory loss
  - Parkinson's disease
  - Cardiovascular disease
  - Diabetes
  - Psoriasis
  - Rheumatoid arthritis

I love DHEA! After 3 days of using DHEA I felt as though my body had been jump started. I had a positive energy shift and I no longer has an afternoon "slump".

<u>Note</u>: If you are under 40 years old, your body is probably making all the DHEA it needs. Do not take DHEA if you have an enlarged prostate or prostate cancer. Do not take if you are pregnant or nursing. Stick to the recommended dose. Some people think "well, I'll take a lot if it's that good." **Normal doses are: Women: 10 – 25 mg. Men: 25 – 50 mg.** Mega doses in women may cause facial hair, acne and/or deepening of the voice. <u>Note</u>: this will cease when DHEA is reduced.

As you pass the age of 40, DHEA can increase and maintain your youthful vigor!
P.S. If you find yourself tired ALL the time, this is an indication of low adrenal function. **See chapter 3.**

"That energy is God's energy, an energy deep within you, God himself willing and working at what will give him the most pleasure."
Philippians 2:13

Chapter 3

Tired Most of the Time? You May Have Adrenal Fatigue

(Known as: *The 21ˢᵗ Century Stress Syndrome*)

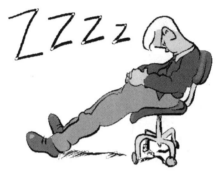

Ask yourself:
Am I tired a lot? This is NOT a symptom of aging.
Are you saying: *"Barbara . . . I'm so tired. I can't act or feel young."*
Well if you wake up tired or feel tired halfway through the day, your adrenal glands probably need a boost. Adrenals that are firing on all cylinders will make you feel 25 years old. I promise!

Adrenal Fatigue is common and growing by leaps & bounds. Perhaps 80% of Americans have some form of adrenal fatigue. No wonder so many of us look and feel lifeless, weary and worn-out. When adrenals are functioning at full strength, you feel energetic, vigorous, and strong.

Adrenals are SO important to keep healthy. Why?
They are necessary for energy production, fat burning and hormone production and, for women especially after menopause.

However, the adrenals are the glands of stress and therefore the first to fail under stressful conditions. Daily stresses add up over time. The adrenals eventually become "exhausted" and stress tolerance declines dramatically. You start to feel your health deteriorating. Think of this as a "leaky boat". You have to "plug the hole" or you will sink!

Back in our mother's day, adrenal fatigue was often called a "Nervous Breakdown". And it could have been fixed! My own mother checked herself into a facility for a week thinking she has a nervous breakdown. Well, she was raising 5 children born within 7 years of each other. Her adrenal glands were exhausted!

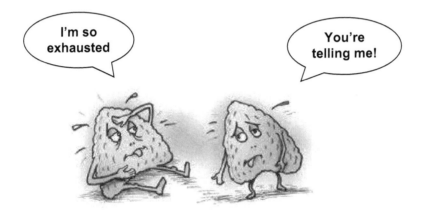

Adrenal Fatigue is nothing new! The first reported cases were seen in 1898 in France following a severe flu epidemic. According to Dr. James Wilson, (whom I call America's Adrenal Doctor), "80% of Americans suffer from Adrenal Fatigue; the other 20% are in denial." However, you and I are not in denial, we are on alert.

I find that adrenal fatigue is often not properly diagnosed or treated. People wander from doctor to doctor looking for help that never comes!

Guess what?
If you have low adrenal function, even treating your hypothyroid will not alleviate all of your symptoms.
As Dr. Wilson Says: At the beginning of adrenal fatigue, the disease is difficult to recognize but EASY to treat.
At the end, the disease is easy to recognize but DIFFICULT to treat.

He says: "All peri-menopausal & menopausal women should be on adrenal supplements for at least 2-4 months"
I also believe all men over the age of 45 should do the same.

Self Test:
If you can say: "After__(event)__I was never the same." It is probable you have had an adrenal onslaught which caused Adrenal Fatigue.

What are the Adrenal Fatigue symptoms?
- You wake up tired
- Crave salt (you have no aldotestosterone, can't maintain your sodium levels)
- Lethargy
- Everything takes more effort, you feel exhausted
- Irritable
- Muscle weakness (due to low cortisol/low testosterone)
- Episodic energy (not consistent)
- Liver spots
- Crave high fat foods
- Crave salt & caffeine
- Feel helpless
- Dry, thin skin
- Hair loss
- Weight gain
- Increased marital discord
- Low libido
- Increased allergies
- Hyperventilation: frequent sighing
- Asthma, frequent colds
- Skin rashes

Adrenal Fatigue Energy Pattern:
- Your best sleep is not at night but 7am-9am
- You feel better after lunch
- 2-4 pm = low feelings
- Around 6 pm you feel the best of the day

Aggravating Factors.
These <u>must</u> change or you will <u>not</u> heal!
- Constant life or work stress
- Poor dietary habits
- Unhappy relationships (work/home)
- Lack of exercise of any type
- Insufficient enjoyable activities
- No control over how you spend your time

<u>Low adrenal function contributes to:</u>
- Fibromyalgia
- Chronic fatigue
- Rheumatoid arthritis
- Lack of libido
- Allergies
- Feeling overwhelmed
- Environmental sensitivities
- Premature menopause
- Auto immune diseases

What To Do?
Adrenal Fatigue Treatment via Lifestyle Changes
- Get sleep: bad sleep & bad adrenals go together. The adrenals repair at night
- Go to bed by 9-9:30 pm
- Try to sleep until 9 am if possible during the rebuilding stage
- No nightly news, no horror movies, no animals in the bed. (sorry, I'm a dog & cat lover, too!)
- Lie down on breaks for 15-30 minutes (at 10 am & between 3-5) if at all possible
- Alleviate the stressful situation (as best you can)
- Laugh (laughter enhances the parapathetic system)

- Chew food really well (30 times per mouthful)
- Don't get out of bed until you think of something pleasant. Really!
- Eliminate "energy suckers" from your life, those people who consistently make you feel stressed or "down"
- Increase protein intake, decrease carbs. (Vegans are difficult to heal from A.F.)
- Eat regular meals. This is VERY helpful. (Email or call for the handout: How To Eat With Adrenal Fatigue)
- No fruit in the morning, concentrate on protein
- Very mild exercise if you can (increases low cortisol, decreases high cortisol)
- Spend some time with a friend
- Take a daily "Joy Break"

Make a "Good for Me" / "Bad for Me" list (2 columns).
In the next 6 months try to concentrate on the "Good For Me" listings. Slowly eliminate the "Bad for Me"
On the adrenal fatigue questionnaire, a score above 40 equals some degree adrenal fatigue
Email or call for a copy of the questionnaire!
877-539-6200 or barbara@askbarbarahoffman.com

Supplements to treat Adrenal Fatigue
Excellent formulas developed by Dr. James Wilson can bring you back to adrenal health.

For mild-moderate Adrenal Fatigue:
- Super Adrenal Stress Formula (Dr. Wilson) –supplies specific vitamins & minerals necessary for energy and adrenal hormone production.
- Adrenal C Formula (Dr. Wilson) – delivers extra vitamin C, trace minerals and bioflavonoids used up during stress, and compensates for metabolic changes that occur during stress.

Separate nutrients:
- Pregnenelone (precursor to adrenal hormones) 25 mg at night
- Phosphatidylserine

For Severe Adrenal Fatigue:
Use these with the other supplements.

- Adrenal Rebuilder™ (Dr. Wilson) – Contains glandular extracts which will heal deplenished adrenals. 6 capsules daily for several months. Severe cases: take for 1 year. Also, for severe cases, you can use actual cortisol (Isocort, Cortef) in addition to the glandulars. After 6 months, you can withdraw the cortisol.

For Children: Crush any of these and put in food. Children respond very well. (An interesting note: Adrenal supplements can actually decrease asthma in children.)

Other Helpful Nutrients:
- Melatonin 3-6 mg at night
- L-Theonine/GABA 200 mg or more (increases alpha brain waves)
- Calming herbal teas: passion flower, lemon balm

Time Frame to Healing Adrenal Fatigue
Mild   6-9 months
Moderate   12-18 months
Severe   12-24 months

The Good News: When healed your gland will stop struggling and you will feel like yourself again!

If you do not wish to purchase a complete formula, here are the separate healing nutrients:
- Niacin 125-150 mg/day
- B6 150 mg/day
- Vitamin C 2000-5000 mg/day
- Vitamin E 800 IU/day
- Calcium 400 mg in the morning
- Magnesium 800 mg in the evening
- Licorice (unless you have high blood pressure) It elevates cortisol levels and keeps receptor sites active

Lab Tests for Cortisol levels

A blood test is not a great way to test for Adrenal Fatigue. The best ways to test are urine and saliva.

You can order your own tests from ZRT laboratories and have the results sent directly to you. Call if you need information for ZRT labs.

Beloveds, this is now an epidemic, even in children. Let's stop it now for you and your family!

I have a college-aged son on a regimen of good adrenal support for the past two years. He definitely notices the difference. My husband and I do not miss a day of our adrenal support. It's too important!

"I can do all things through Christ which strengthens me."
Philippians 4:13

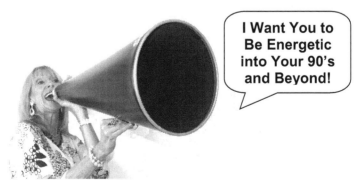

I Want You to Be Energetic into Your 90's and Beyond!

Chapter 4

No Anxiety For The Younger You

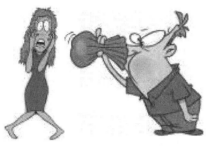

Anxiety makes us look old.
Anxiety and the stress of always fretting can age us quickly.
We look fearful, frail, and haggard when we are anxious. If you are anxious, you will not be your best 'Young You'

Here is an email I received that is very typical of many others. Read it and see if you can relate:

"Dear Barbara:
Can you help me? About 2 years ago I started to get increasingly anxious, right around when I started into perimenopause and skipping periods. My body started feeling like I was jumping out of my skin. Then I would start worrying about every little thing. Then I got crabby at my husband and kids and everyone wanted to avoid Mom. Now I feel it is getting worse. If I go to the grocery store I can feel panicky in the store and sometimes I am too anxious to even think about what I want to buy. I have NO reason to be so anxious and I feel it is something wrong with my hormones. Nothing like this runs in my family and my sisters keep telling me to calm down, but that is not easy. I refuse to take anxiety medications because I am afraid of them and I think this is something I can help. What can I do? I'm so tired of being nervous & anxious."

If YOU have been anxious, you know the symptoms: irrational or intense fear, muscle tension, jaw-clenching, teeth-grinding, insomnia, restlessness, nervousness, a choking sensation or nausea, jumpiness, irritability, shakiness, sudden sweating, pulling on your hair....you may have some of these or all.

Mild to moderate anxiety or generalized anxiety is extremely widespread and common. Even people who say they were never anxious before in their lives can develop anxiety and/or panic attacks as they experience hormonal changes. It is ESPECIALLY common for women during peri-menopause. As a matter of fact, it can be the first sign that you are entering this phase.

Women: Other periods of hormonal change that can trigger anxiety in women are: Puberty, PMS, and following childbirth.

I did not have any post-partum depression, but I definitely had post-partum anxiety. I was absolutely convinced that if I lay my baby down, something awful was going to happen when I was not looking. It was both irrational and intense at the same time! Hysterectomy can also cause anxiety due to the dramatic decrease of hormones that ensues.

Men: Anxiety can seem to "come out nowhere" as your hormones become unbalanced and GABA declines in your brain. Medication for anxiety is prescribed freely. In fact, women who simply complain of hot flashes are often given Xanax, Ativan or Valium. Men are often given Atvan with no discussion about what might be causing the anxiety.

Our email writer is afraid to take anti-anxiety meds and she has a valid point for women AND men. These medications can be highly addictive and do not correct the root cause of the anxiety. They simply mask the symptoms so that you can function. Also, it has been found that these drugs can actually make symptoms worse. Many say they will feel calm, but also like a "zombie" while taking them. There are ways that you can naturally reduce or eliminate your symptoms.
Let's look at the main types of anxiety.

Hormonal Anxiety In Women

If the progesterone/estrogen ratio is low, anxiety can ensue. Progesterone is known to enhance the calming effect of GABA (gamma-aminobutyric acid) by activating the GABA receptor sites and it also suppresses the brain's excitatory response.

The anti-anxiety affect has been noticed very quickly in some people with reports of as little as ten minutes. The anti-anxiety response has been compared to that found with benzodiazepine drugs, but without the risk of addiction. Isn't that wonderful?

GABA in itself is a calming neurotransmitter. If progesterone & GABA are used together the calming effect is enhanced. The recommended dose of progesterone is between 40–80 mg per day. You can use more during an anxious episode.

"Is It In Your Head" Anxiety – Women & Men

For years, people, mostly women, have been told that their anxiety is "all in their head". Guess what? This is not entirely untrue! If your neurotransmitters are not balanced, your brain makes you more prone to a high level of excitability and more prone to a fearful response to events. Constant high levels of the excitatory neurotransmitters (adrenaline, epinephrine) and low levels of the calming neurotransmitters (GABA and serotonin) can alter the circuitry of the brain. Your stress response never recedes keeping you in a chronic state of adrenalin-fueled feelings and behavior.
In other words, a "nervous wreck!"

The messages from the brain are designed to be sent in a calm, rhythmic fashion. When the neurotransmitter balance is disrupted the signals are sent in a jerky fashion and often too many at once. Your entire body feels restless, your heart can be beating faster, emotions are heightened, mental focus becomes very narrow, you can't breathe deeply and you can experience sheer panic. You will definitely have problems sleeping as well.
This can be helped! There are literally thousands and thousands of people in your shoes. Do NOT feel alone!

What are the natural recommendations for anxiety?
- **GABA:** Involved in the production of endorphins, the brain chemicals that create a feeling of well- being.
- **L-Theonine:** A naturally occurring amino acid found in green tea. It is involved in the formation of GABA
- **5-HTP:** Raises serotonin levels which promotes a sense of calm focus.
- **Vitamin B12 & Folic Acid:** I especially like Rodex Forte or a sublingual Vitamin B-12
- **Melatonin:** Good sleep promotes good brain chemistry.

These supplements work to calm you without drowsiness and will also increase mental clarity. GABA and L-Theonine seem to work the fastest. I love a product called Zen-Mind. It worked wonders for me!

Of course, if you have a severe anxiety disorder, including OCD, post-traumatic stress disorder or social phobias, you should contact your healthcare practitioner. However, these conditions afflict only a small minority of people who suffer from anxiety. The rest of you might want to give GABA and progesterone a try. You could add the other supplements as needed. You can be DELIVERED!

"Be anxious for nothing, but in everything by prayer and supplication with thanksgiving let your requests be made known to God. And the peace of God, which surpasses all comprehension, shall guard your hearts and your minds in Christ Jesus."
Philippians 4:6-7

Don't Let Anxiety Age YOU! Take Action!

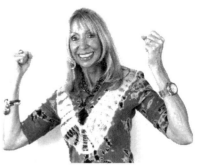

Chapter 5

Depression, Be Gone! The Younger You Will NOT Be Blue

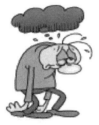

How do depressed people look?
Sad, dreary, careworn and older than their years. When your brain is nourished and balanced, you will look vibrant, youthful and healthy.

Are you feeling depressed?
Are you tired of taking antidepressants?
Do you wonder: Am I really depressed or am I just hooked on antidepressants?
Are these drugs really the solution for me?
Do you wake up feeling bleak and pessimistic rather than exuberant and light-hearted? No wonder you feel old.
I deeply relate to this topic. I have talked to so many people all over the United States and actually over the world, and depression has become almost epidemic. Many of you, men and women, have ended up taking antidepressant drugs.
As a matter of fact, there is a specific drug that became a $2.66-billion industry in the United States alone.

I notice in my experiences with people all over, especially in the U.S., that if you go to a doctor and tell him or her that you feel depressed you will most likely receive a prescription for an anti-depressant.
I know because it happened to me in 2008.

Mild depressive symptoms ebb and flow. Major depressive symptoms spiral downward. You keep going down, down, down.

There is never any ebb. You are never having a glimmer of light and you can get very dark thoughts, and for those people prescription drugs can be extremely important. However, much of the depression in women over the age of 20 is hormonal and can be helped with hormone balance. I saw something very poignant about three months ago. Former Chief of Staff Karl Rove was on a major talk show, and he was talking about his mother who committed suicide when she was in her 40s. And the interviewer said, "Well, Karl what do you think happened?" And he looked at the interviewer and he said, "I don't know. I think she just didn't have any hope." Think about it.

She was young, she was in her 40s.

What if that was hormonal and could have been helped? That is truly tragic.

There is Hope For Your Hormones, the name of my radio show, YouTube channel, and blog.

You could be feeling depressed because your hormones are low or your serotonin levels are low or both!

You are not alone if you are suffering from depression, but, ironically, that is one of the isolating factors. You think you ARE alone which makes you feel worse. Guess what? The World Health Organization estimates that 5% to 10% of the entire population is depressed at any given moment. So, the moment that you are depressed, 10% of the rest of the people in the world are also going through depression. Does that mean we all need to be on a potent antidepressant drug? Could it be that environmental toxins, the way we eat, and our stress are causing it? If that is what it is, it can be helped naturally.

Here is how it seems to work: you don't feel right, something is off, you don't have your joy for life, you feel that when you get up in the morning you do not have the energy to even face the day.

For women, you are crying at the slightest thing, for no real reason. You just want this feeling to end and if you are told a pill will help, you take the pill.

This is a story that might help you. My sister, who had turned 50, called me and said, "Barb I just can't get going anymore. I have lost it. I think I am just getting old and I am tired of life. I am so depressed." She was only 50 years old. She is a baby in God's eyes. I said, "It may be that you need to get your hormones adjusted." She lives in New York and she made an appointment to see a doctor about her hormones. She told the doctor that she was depressed and she thought it was her hormones. She called me when she came home, and guess what? She was given a choice of Effexor or Lexapro. And I said, "Well, what about your hormones?" She said "He did not mention anything about them, I guess I will try these pills. I went to the drug store and I filled them." So, this is the mindset of the medical community: the doctor has a person in front of him or her who is feeling depressed, not feeling right, no zest for life. They want to fix it. They do want to help you, but the first line of defense in many cases is to give the antidepressant. Why else would this industry be so prosperous? My sister took the pills for a year. She was in New York, I am in California, and I am putting cold compresses on my head that my sister is on antidepressants for what I believe is hormone imbalance. Eventually, she got tired of them; said she felt like a zombie, tired all the time. She finally got on bio-identical hormones and she got better!

There is also an area of controversy as to whether antidepressant drugs really work for mild to moderate depression. Many studies have been done that show that antidepressant drugs are no better than a placebo in these cases. You can find these studies yourself on the internet.

The Serotonin Factor:
It is common knowledge that people who are depressed most often have low levels of serotonin. The symptoms of low serotonin are depression, impatience, short attention span, craving sweets and high carb foods, and insomnia.

The vast majority of antidepressants are called SSRIs; drugs which help to keep the serotonin levels that you already have in your brain active. It recycles them. So, you keep going round and round with the same serotonin that you already have. The drugs do not do anything to raise the serotonin levels, but they do keep your serotonin at a somewhat even keel.

Here are the common side effects of an SSRI anti-depressant: Nausea, headaches, anxiety, nervousness, insomnia, drowsiness, diarrhea, dry mouth, loss of appetite, sweating, tremor, and rash. A very, very common side effect which is not often told to you prior to being given the drug is WEIGHT GAIN! I believe that the reason we are not told is that women would then not take the prescription. Many would say, "I'd rather be depressed than gain 20 pounds." Maybe men, too. The most popular drugs, in case you do not know if your drug is an antidepressant are Prozac, Celexa, Paxil, Lexapro, Zoloft, Effexor, Cymbalta, and Wellbutrin. However, if the reason you're depressed is low serotonin levels, you can boost that naturally!

There is a supplement (natural) called 5-HTP, (5-hydroxytryptophan) which has been shown to produce significant benefits for depression. It is also good, by the way, for weight loss, headaches, and fibromyalgia. The recommended starting dose is 50 mg one to three times per day. If you are already on an antidepressant, you cannot just add 5-HTP because you can get what is called "serotonin poisoning" wherein serotonin levels become too high. So, you would have to wean off your antidepressant according to your doctor's instructions. If you are not already taking an antidepressant, you can take 5-HTP.

DHEA:
New research shows that the hormonal supplement DHEA can help relieve mild to moderate depression in middle age individuals. A study with DHEA treatment resulted in a 50% reduction in depression symptoms in half of the participants. Researchers observed that in "in 50% of depressed outpatients who do not respond to first-line antidepressant

treatments, or those unwilling to take traditional antidepressants, DHEA may have a useful role in the treatment of mild to moderate severe midlife-onset major and minor depression." People, 50% is a good number of people who can be helped.

What Else Is Good?
Essential fatty acids are proven to help depression. L-Theanine is also proven to help depression and that is found in green tea. Another step you could take to lift your spirits is to eliminate sugar! And another supplement that is very, very good is called St. John's Wort. In Germany, doctors give St. John's Wort out for depression eight times more frequently than Prozac. As a matter of fact, several double-blinds studies have shown it is more effective for moderate cases of depression. SAM-e is also excellent for depression. For depression coupled with anxiety, GABA can be very helpful. Also, increasing the protein in your diet can alleviate depression!

Testosterone is found to be good for men who are depressed. DHEA is also good for the men.

What Else?
Here are a couple of other things that you can do. Stop and do something enjoyable. I want you to do some mild exercise, even if you just walk. I'm a naturopath; I'm probably supposed to be out there with those medicine balls and those free weights and the treadmill. Instead, I just walk. So, let's just get outside and walk. You can go to a movie. One of the most fun things I did when I actually went through depression: I went to a ball game. I put on a T-shirt and jeans, a little ball cap, and I went and sat in the stands and cheered on the home team, and I tell you, that was like a tonic. I really felt better after that. How about church? How about a women's group? I joined a book club. I mean that was fun. My assignment was to read. Well, that was fun, to have that as your assignment! Then I went and sat and talked about the book with other ladies and it was cheerful and inexpensive. I did it at the local senior center and it was perfect for me.

Here's another important thing. *Give it time.* Expect your mood to improve gradually, not immediately. Feeling better takes time. Take the pressure off yourself. Find a way to have your needs accommodated by people around you. You shouldn't feel that you have to do everything for everybody. When you have your hormones & neurotransmitters balanced and good serotonin levels, you will be able to walk through life beaming, luminous and inspiring to others. A younger you!

"Even when the way goes through Death Valley,
I'm not afraid when you walk at my side.
Your trusty shepherd's crook makes me feel secure."
Psalm 23:4

Chapter 6

HELP! My Sex Drive Drove Away!

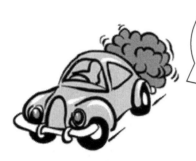

No, I haven't found my libido yet. BUT I do know it's not at the office, the bank, the grocery store or the drycleaners.

You may have chuckled when you read this heading, but a lady really said this to me and she was in tears. This lady said, "I love my husband with all my heart; I believe God gave him to me and I really want him to be happy, but I just cannot muster up any desire and I feel so bad. I pretend to be asleep so he just won't touch me. I'm so disappointed in myself".

Wow! I wish I had the exact count of how many women have asked this question – probably 50,000 over the years, if not more. So, even if this is something you don't talk about to your friends, please know you are NOT alone!

I think men would be surprised to see how sad women are about this issue. Perhaps they think women are just being selfish. This is NOT true. I see and hear that there is a great deal of pain involved. For both sexes, libido is not something that can easily be summoned on command and it is not easy to talk yourself into having desire. You can totally adore your husband or wife and think they are an absolute gift from God and still not be able to "gettin the mood."

What can you do?

Guess What?

In almost every case, IT IS NOT YOUR FAULT!
Researchers estimate that 50% of all women aged 20-65 have experienced low libido and I know this is true…it may be more if you count temporary episodes. Men over the age of 45 also frequently report cases of diminished sexual desire. They are usually more disturbed by this than the women because now they don't feel "manly". What's going on? Libido can be psychological, but there are many physiologic body factors that can be overcome to put YOU on the road to restoration.

Road Blocks on the Libido Highway:

- Hormone imbalance
- Fatigue
- Stress
- Anxiety / Anxiety Medications
- Depression
- Women Only:
- Hot flashes (make it difficult to feel sexy)
- Vaginal Dryness (which can easily be helped)
- Hysterectomy…starting on synthetic hormones
- Birth Control Pill (which lower testosterone levels)

New Drugs on the Horizon?

We all know about Viagra for you men – the blue pill, which is heavily promoted on television and in print. However, Viagra has side effects which include headaches, stomach pain, nasal congestion, nausea, diarrhea, loss of hearing, ringing in the ears and dizziness.

Well, it was inevitable….Pharmaceutical companies developed a "Little Pink Pill" which was supposed to be the female counterpart to Viagra.

However, in June, 2010 the FDA said "no" because the benefits of the drug did not outweigh the side effects.

What was the "Little Pink Pill" supposed to do? Raise serotonin levels and dopamine levels. Well, guess what? You can do that with the supplements 5-HTP and L-Tyrosine.

How Can You Improve Libido Naturally So Your Sex Drive can make a "U-Turn"

Natural Progesterone for Women & Men
Women:
Low libido has usually been associated with menopause, but it is still very common among relatively young women. Many women have a normal menstrual period indicating the presence of sufficient estrogen, yet still have low libido. This is due to low progesterone levels or a low progesterone-to-estrogen ration.
At ovulation, progesterone levels rise and sexual drive is heightened. This is meant to ensure that a woman will be receptive to procreation. Remember, progesterone is called the *"Feel Good"* Hormone.

Older, non-ovulating women often have the uncomfortable symptoms of hot flashes, night sweats, depression or anxiety, and vaginal dryness. Who would be in the mood when feeling depressed, bloated and irritable? Progesterone can help!
As I have talked to women who have been on progesterone crème, I have learned that their low libido had been <u>restored</u> in about 3 months of use, sometimes less. The woman who told me "My sex drive drove off" called and said "It drove back!" There are so many wonderful testimonials from very happy women. The men often call, too. One man brought his wife a year's supply of crème, saying "I'm never going to let her run out of this stuff". He speaks for many!

Men:
A man's wonderful libido-enhancing testosterone can begin converting to a form called DHT, di-hydro-testosterone. Instead of feeling manly & virile, they begin to feel moody, fatigued, and often gain weight and become listless and uninterested in having fun with their spouse. It's hormonal and NOT your fault. Progesterone can stop the conversion of testosterone to DHT (which also helps prevent prostate problems and male pattern baldness, by the way).

God designed you to have "Vim &Vigor" all the days of your life. Remember the men in the Bible!
A good dose of progesterone for Women: 40 mg / day
A good dose of progesterone for Men: 10 – 20 mg / day

Testosterone? It's prescription-only. Try DHEA instead!
Until recently, doctors were very willing to prescribe
testosterone for women to improve libido. This treatment has
now been discredited not only because of the masculinizing
effects of testosterone, but because testosterone has been
shown to contribute to liver damage if used at too high a
strength or for too long a period. If you do receive a
prescription for testosterone, the common dose for women is
2%. If you are looking for bio-identical testosterone, be careful
with the synthetic drug Estratest, it contains a synthetic form of
testosterone called methyl-testosterone. I believe that the best
testosterone is a bio-identical cream form made by a
compounding pharmacy. For men, if testosterone is indicated,
the gel or the patch seems to work the best.

Great News! DHEA has been proven to increase testosterone
levels, so this is a good choice. As an added bonus,
supplementing with DHEA increases energy and helps burn
"belly" fat! Now, that's my kind of supplement! For women, it
can also reduce vaginal atrophy. Men who take DHEA report
feeling more amorous. Some men have said that they feel an
increase in libido about 30 minutes after an evening dose.
Recommended DHEA dose for women: 10–20 mg / day
Recommended DHEA dose for men: 25–50 mg / day

Tribulus Terrestris
Tribulus Terrestris has been used by body-builders for
decades. Studies have shown that Tribulus taken for just 5
days increased testosterone levels. It appears to trigger the
release of LH which sends a message to cells to produce
more testosterone. In women, Tribulus has also had a
favorable effect on loss of interest in sex. Results will not be
immediate in women…you should allow 40-50 days for effects
to be noticed. Other positive changes: Increase in muscle
tone (without increase in exercise). How about THAT?
I like a product called Testron SX.
Recommended dose for women: 750 mg /day
Recommended dose for men: 750 mg / twice a day

Avena Sativa "Wild Oats"

This little product is considered by many researchers to be a true aphrodisiac for both women and men. It appears to contain substances that have a similar makeup to natural testosterone and works very well in men for both sexual energy and strength of erections. Some women who take Avena Sativa report that libido increases "dramatically" and yet others will not note an increase.

So, this is a supplement you would need to try for yourself. Fortunately, it's not expensive. Also, a very interesting benefit is that takers have reported that Avena has reduced their cravings for sweets. (But NOT their sweetie!)

Recommended dose for men & women: 750 mg (1 tablet) 1–3 times daily.

L-Tyrosine

Studies have shown that L-tyrosine (an amino acid) increases the rate at which the brain produces dopamine…just what the "Little Pink Pill" was going to do and it is NATURAL to the body. Increased dopamine is associated with higher libido. I love this supplement! It also suppresses appetite and elevates mood and "feelings of joy". My husband and I take it daily!

Recommended dose: 500 mg, 1 – 3 times per day.

L-Arginine

For men, it has been called an herbal alternative to Viagra and is recommended by many physicians for erectile dysfunction. Men who take it report improvement in erectile function. It has also been found to help increase sperm count if that is of interest to you.

Women have reported increased sensitivity and lubrication leading to enhancement of libido.

Recommended dose: 500 mg. 1 – 3 times per day.

Libido can be helped NATURALLY!

The feelings of desire can come back. Do not give up! Also, be generous in spirit toward your partner. God loves a cheerful giver! You are also protecting your assets….that is YOUR husband (or YOUR wife).

I once had someone ask my husband's secretary if he was married. His secretary said "yes, he is married" and the woman asked "How married is he?" Imagine!
Let me tell you….
I want my husband to feel VERY married! Sometimes just participating can be sexy in itself.

Also, remember that if one person wants more sex and the other wants less….the "less" person has the power. Giving up that power can actually be a joyful feeling. And for more joy feelings, remember
L-Tyrosine. And one final tip….for weight loss…Grab your Mate instead of Your Plate!
Libido is not a simple subject, but it is important and I absolutely believe that libido can be restored. I want to help you.
I know things change and change is not bad.
Your sex drive may come back in a more mature manner; different than those overwhelming hormonal feelings of youth. You are wiser now and your body has undergone some changes.
But we can still feel young and vibrant! Let's do our best to keep the intimacy alive for our partner.
Call me if you need more help. I have more comprehensive handouts on all of the wonderful products I mentioned.

Let Your Sex Drive Make Its U-Turn!
Feel youthful & vibrant like you did in your 30's.

"Let thy fountain be blessed: and rejoice with the wife (or husband, my words) *of thy youth."*
Proverbs 5:18-19

Chapter 7

Younger Brain, Younger You

Learn How to Have a *Young, Healthy & Vibrant Brain*
Restore Your Remarkable Memory!

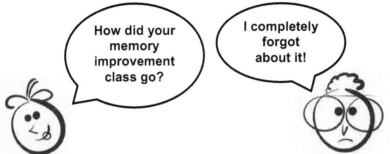

Oh dear, what has happened to us?
Why can't we remember things the way we used to?
Is this an inevitable part of aging? No! Our brains have been assaulted by environmental toxins and stress which affects our memory, focus, and mental clarity. Our brains are a magnificent data base that contain information attained throughout our lives. It's all there. Often, we just can't access the information. We need some brain-boosters

You can prevent:
- Cognitive Decline
- Dementia
- Alzheimers

I want to teach you how!

The 5 Worst Enemies of a Healthy Brain
- Toxins
- Stress
- Sleep Deprivation
- Poor Nutrition
- Lack of Sun

What Is The Best Anti-Aging Approach?

You must maintain your levels of:
- Dopamine
- Serotonin
- Phosphatidylserine
- Progesterone

Stress Reduction is Crucial
- Extreme stress will immediately reduce memory & cognition by at least 50% as stress disengages the frontal lobe.
- Serotonin and GABA are significantly depleted by a high stress life. Cortisol sucks up serotonin like a vacuum cleaner. You need Serotonin & GABA to feel good!
- Don't let Glutamate take over your brain (excitatory response). It causes inflammatory pain, dementia, stroke, anxiety, and even alcohol dependency. It damages your brain. Balance with GABA!

Support Your Neurotransmitters To Feel And Look Younger!

What Do I Need?

Dopamine: A vital component of brain health. It helps the positive transmission of signals. The human brain has 5 known types of dopamine receptors. Dopamine contributes to our ability to learn, our working memory and our attention span. Low dopamine can lead to Parkinson's disease, and ADHD. Dopamine is necessary for feelings of joy and increases focus.

Raise Your Dopamine Naturally with:
- L-Tyrosine 500-1000 mg/day

Serotonin: Low serotonin can lead to forgetfulness, feelings of being "scatter-brained" and feeling "worn out". No wonder we feel old!

Raise Your Serotonin Naturally with:
- 7 hours of Sleep per night (or serotonin will drop)
- Progesterone 40-80 mg/day
- 5-HTP 50-100 mg/day
- Melatonin 3 mg/day

Phosphatidlyserine
PS promotes brain function, brain repair, memory & cognition.
- Best nutritional support on the market for memory according to brain researchers!
- Increases neuronal membrane fluidity (cell-to-cell communication)
- Excellent for those 50 or older – can prevent dementia & possibly Alzheimer's disease
- Improves memory loss due to aging
- Improves cognition
- Helps the brain retrieve information
- Also, excellent for stress reduction

I find that after only 2 weeks on PS, users report a marked difference in their ability to: remember and focus. People say they actually feel their intelligence returning & expanding. This is one of my all-time favorites! Results are cumulative. After 3 months on PS I was remembering things from when I was 5 years old. I actually remembered my first day in Kindergarten. **Recommended dose:** 100 mg twice daily for 1 month. Then, for maintenance, take 100 mg once daily.

The brain is greatly affected by the delicate balance of neurotransmitters and hormones.
Progesterone is a natural neuro-protectant.

Progesterone
Benefits of Progesterone for the Brain:
- Enhances and nourishes GABA receptor sites
- Helps eliminate brain fog
- Regulates cognition, mood, & brain regeneration
- May improve outcomes from traumatic brain injury, including stroke

In Conclusion:
Supplements are vitally important!

Experts agree supplementation is necessary. We cannot always get the proper nutrients from our food!
Supplements increase **brain power and speed.**

Other Tips:
- Green Tea – Contains L-Theanine and antioxidants which enhance memory
- Eat Walnuts! Walnuts contain DHA (the omega-3 that the brain loves)

To fight a disease after it has occurred is like trying to dig a well when one is thirsty.
Act Preventively!

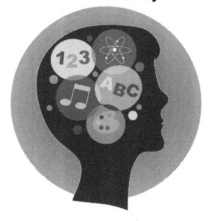

"For God did not give us a spirit of fear, but of power and of love and of a sound mind!"
Second Timothy 1:7

Chapter 8

Hair Loss / Thinning Hair

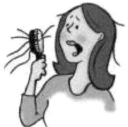

We are extremely attached to our hair. Of course! We have had it since we were babies. If you are over 45 and experiencing hair loss, you are not alone. Two thirds of all women & men over the age of 45 experience hair loss. Why? Most of it is hormonal. When estrogen and progesterone levels get low, we begin losing hair. For men, when testosterone begins converting to DHT (dihydrotestosterone) you lose hair.

Hormones?
How can you tell if it is indeed hormonal? Hair loss due to hormonal imbalance tends to start at the crown and is diffuse instead of bald patches. If this is you, I have good news! It can be corrected with progesterone. When progesterone and estrogen levels fall, your androgens (male hormones) dominate. Testosterone is one of these androgens that become dominant. It combines with an enzyme and forms DHT, dihydrotestosterone, which causes your follicles to go into a resting phase. The hair coming out of the follicle becomes thinner and thinner with each cycle. Finally, without any intervention on your part, the follicle closes up and produces no new hairs.

Stress?
Hair loss also occurs as a result of stress. If you experience frequent or chronic stress, your adrenal glands stop producing their essential hormones and you get adrenal-stress-related hair loss.

Hair loss of this type is usually on your head only and is a result of both low estrogen and progesterone and high levels of adrenal stress. A good adrenal support is needed for you. (See Chapter 3) I believe Rhodiola is also a must for you.

Thyroid?
Your hair loss could also be related to thyroid problems. If you experience hair loss all over your body, including your armpits and pubic area, then it is usually thyroid related. However, be careful which thyroid medication you receive. One of the listed side effects of Synthroid is hair loss. How ironic is that? Ask for bio-identical thyroid hormone.

There Is Help!
To sum it up, hair loss is not just genetic. As I said, it is commonly a result of hormone imbalance. Many women experience hair loss during pregnancy, post-birth, menopause, and peri-menopause when hormones levels are fluctuating. For both sexes, hair loss can also be caused by adrenal dysfunction, Vitamin B-12 deficiency, low protein, low essential fatty acids (70% of us do not have sufficient essential fatty acids in our blood streams), and the use of anti-cholestrol drugs (statins), antidepressants, and birth control. Anorexia and bulimia also cause hair loss.

What can be done? A doctor might recommend Rogaine, which contains Minoxidil. Minoxidil is a synthetic drug that works by re-stimulating your follicles.

If you are looking for natural treatments, here they are:
1. **Progesterone** – to prevent DHT formation
2. **Bio-identical Estrogen (women)** – If you're experiencing hair growth on your face, you might need some estrogen. Make sure it is bio-identical.
3. **Cortisol or Adrenal Support Formulas** – If you experience moderate-high stress, then these are great for you.
4. **Vitamin B-6 and B-12** – My favorite product is called Rodex Forte and it is also found to reverse the graying of hair. YES!

5. **L-Tyrosine** – L-Tyrosine nourishes the thyroid gland to prevent thyroid-related hair loss. Don't wait for a thyroid crisis to take care of this important gland.
6. **Essential Fatty Acids**
7. **Vitamin E**

Take Heart

Hair is adaptive. Those follicles can be restored. Your instinct is to be gentle with your hair when you wash it, but you want to stimulate those follicles. Give yourself a nice head massage or buy a stimulating shampoo. A good one that I like is called Chinese Herbs Regenerating Scalp Serum that contains apple stem cells.

Thin hair runs in my family, but I did something about it! I don't think there's a single follicle on my head that has not been stimulated. I rarely lose any hair at all. I believe my progesterone crème and L-Tyrosine are responsible. You don't have to experience hair loss either.

Hair loss runs in the family? Genetics are not the entire story. You can take important steps to prevent and reverse thinning hair. Don't wait!

For hair treatment tips, see Part II – Chapter 23.

"But even the very hairs of your head are all numbered. Fear not therefore: ye are of more value than many sparrows."
Luke 12:7

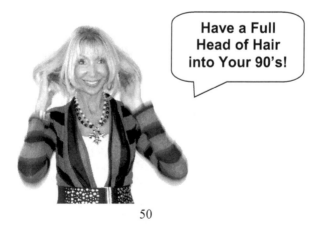

Have a Full Head of Hair into Your 90's!

Chapter 9

Weight Gain – Tame Those Carbs!

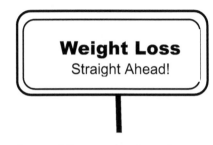

Weight Loss
Straight Ahead!

Have you gained over 10 pounds since the age of 40?
Is it mostly focused around your mid-section?
I like to call these villains "Frankencarbs" because they will have a monstrous effect on your body.
Simple carbs are the culprit.

I have written an entire book on this topic, *Eat Yourself Slender*. But here is the shortened version.

When we eat the wrong carbs, we are chronically elevating insulin levels. This causes chronic accumulation of fat in your fat tissue which becomes very difficult to lose.

"There is something about carbohydrates that allows the consumption of enormous quantities of food (up to 2000 calories) and yet still induces hunger as night approaches". From Good Calories, Bad Calories. Gary Taubes, 2007.
I agree!

If you chronically elevate your blood sugar with carbohydrates and sugar, your body has no choice but to release insulin to take care of the sugar.
The fat cells of adipose tissue are extremely sensitive to insulin compared to other tissues in the body.
Too much insulin tells your body to store fat!

FACT: Obese people favor carbohydrates. They do not appear to eat more calories than lean people, **they eat more carbs.**

Beware of The 23 Worst "FrankenCarbs"

1. Fancy coffee drinks
2. Bagels
3. Waffles / pancakes
4. Potato chips / tortilla chips
5. Most bread
6. Muffins
7. Juice drinks & smoothies
8. Baked goods at coffee shops
9. Yogurt with fruit on the bottom
10. Pretzels
11. Sugary jelly / jam
12. Movie theater popcorn
13. Cheese crackers
14. Ramen noodles
15. Soda
16. Instant oatmeal
17. White flour
18. White rice
19. English muffins
20. Cheese cake
21. Cookies
22. Cake / pie
23. Cereal

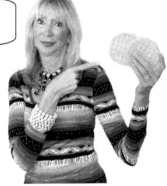

Simple Carbs Are The Culprit!

My Guidelines On How To

Beat the Franken carbs

1. Sugar is the Enemy: It is toxic way beyond its calories

SUGAR IS NOT YOUR FRIEND and it is very addictive. Sugar will turn into FAT in your body, raise your cholesterol and raise your triglycerides. You can lower both by eliminating / cutting down on sugar.

How?

Carbs turn into sugar when you eat them. Yes, that's right! S-U-G-A-R. All carbs will do this, some more slowly than others but the result is the same. Complex carbs found in bread, grains are slower BUT STILL TURN TO SUGAR. Simple carbs such as those found in refined sugar turn quickly, so do the carbs in starches like rice and pasta. And believe it, fructose from fruit also turns to sugar. If you chronically eat too many carbs, you will become insulin resistant. You have to give up sugar and carbs so your body will start to BURN FAT. Then, your body will seek the glucose it needs in the fat storage areas. You will see yourself start to lose the weight! Please try it for 2 weeks and see how good you will feel in addition to losing pounds! I promise!

SHOCKER:

Four grams of sugar in a product = 1 Level teaspoons of white sugar

A lunch that contains 40 grams of sugar is equivalent to eating 10 TEASPOONS OF SUGAR. Most fast food meals will contain this degree of sugar. You might as well just pull out the sugar bowl and eat directly out of it.

How's that for an image? As your insulin levels rise you will be hungrier and hungrier and crave more sugary foods. And your body stores the extra as FAT.

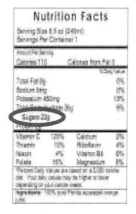

SUGAR IS EVERYWHERE
READ THOSE LABELS!

When you first try to give up sugar, it can almost be painful if your body is addicted. You will crave it! But you can circumvent this.

Note: There are really good supplements discussed in chapter 13 that will help with this.

2. Avoid White Carbohydrates.
The Whiter the Food, The Fatter You Will Get
"The more bread, the sooner dead."
Specifically these "white carbs" are:
- Bread
- Rice
- Cereal
- Potatoes
- Pasta
- Tortillas
- Any breaded fried foods

3. Start Your Day With Protein – Every Day!
Protein, protein, protein. It is almost impossible to overeat protein, so don't worry. Are you eating toast for breakfast? Please stop! The usual 2 slices of toast converts to about 6 teaspoons of sugar! No more cereal, bagels, or even oatmeal in most cases unless you are putting protein powder in it. For most commercial cereals, you would do better if you threw away the cereal and ate the box!

Change Your Breakfast! This one simple step can change your weight and your life.

The Good News:
Protein improves insulin levels.

Protein is burned for energy and NOT stored as fat as carbs are. Protein curbs hunger so you do not overeat and snack too much between meals. Protein takes longer to break down in your body and keeps you satisfied longer. Researchers in France found that high-carb snackers got hungry JUST AS QUICKLY as people who had NO SNACKS AT ALL. Those who snacked on chicken (protein) stayed full almost 40 minutes longer. Now, that is significant!

YOU NEED PROTEIN WITH EVERY MEAL!

Protein causes the brain to produce dopamine, which gives you energy and focus. Protein also helps boost your metabolism. A study from Purdue University showed that people who ate 30% of their calories from protein lost more weight than those who ate only 18%. Protein is important!

4. Eat Repetitiously
Eat the same meals over and over. There are about 50,000 products in an average grocery store. Most will make you fat. Pick 5 meals and repeat them. If you eat out, substitute a salad or veggies in place of potatoes or rice. Tell the waiter you are on a Special Diet. It's the Younger You diet.
You are on the "I won't be fat a minute longer diet". By the way, the true definition of diet comes from the Greek word "diaita" meaning lifestyle, NOT deprivation!

5. Eat 4 times per day
- Breakfast
- Lunch
- Afternoon smaller lunch. Calling this "lunch" will help you avoid snack foods
- Dinner

6. Never Drink Your Calories
a. No fruit juice
b. No soy milk
c. No soft drinks – who needs these, anyway?
Drink: tea, coffee, sparkling water and water

7. Be careful with fruit.
Fructose is a simple sugar.
Fruit contains fructose which, believe it or not, can be fattening. I know many menopausal women in particular who will gain weight the day after they eat too much fruit.
I tested it on myself and a day after I ate nectarines and melon and a pear (all good, right?) I gained 1.5 pounds. WOW! Who knew? So be careful with fruit. Think about it….fruit used to be seasonal and our ancestors just ate what was in season. Now we have so much available that we eat all fruit all the time. For myself, upon experimenting, I have found that I am okay with blueberries, cherries, and apples. Do your own experiment to find your good fruits that will not store as fat.

Note: 1 cup of grapes will turn into about 6 teaspoons of sugar in your body. A banana? 4 teaspoons. The lowest amount of sugar is found in oranges, peaches, and berries.

8. Take a 1 day break every week
Mine is Sunday. Eat whatever you want this day. After a few weeks you will find you don't want to eat unhealthy on your "day off".

9. No Low-Fat Dieting! Fat–Free Is Not Good!
Food manufacturers simply substitute sugar for the fat to restore some of the taste. When you eat a low-fat diet, your intake of carbs increases, causing high levels of sugar. This excess sugar is converted to triglycerides and is stored as fat. Years of a low fat diet results in shrinking of muscle mass, less dense bones, increased blood pressure, increased cholesterol and WEIGHT GAIN. You NEED fats, you do not need sugar.

10. Never Let Yourself Get Too Hungry

When you eat this way, you will not be hungry. If you do feel hungry, you did not eat enough for your breakfast, lunch or dinner.

So eat some more! But eliminate sugar or starch.

You will not gain weight. Right now as I am writing, I feel hungry and it is just 2 pm. I am fixing myself a hardboiled egg (great snack, so keep on hand). I mixed it with some Thousand Island Dressing, some lemon pepper and smushed it up in a little bowl. Yummy and so filling. It will all burn off and not be stored!

11. Legumes Are Your New Best friend

- Canned beans & lentils are fine. Rinse & drain.
- Experiment with red, black, pinto beans, etc.
- Add spices/ vinegar/ hot sauce
- Make fake mashed potatoes. Put a little olive oil in a pan. Heat. Add a can of white kidney beans & mash with a spoon. You can add some water or chicken broth to get the desired consistency. Add salt, pepper, garlic powder, even butter and parmesan cheese. Tastes GREAT! You can also do this with steamed cauliflower. Yummy!
- Mix lentils or beans with some steamed veggies and salsa. Top with some protein like chicken or left-over beef, you can even add avocado. This tastes like a burrito without the tortilla. Delicious!

12. Avocados Are Good For You. Why?

- 60% more potassium than bananas
- Prevent stroke
- Lower cholesterol
- Contain 75% insoluble fiber, the best kind

Barbara's Food Rules

1. Eat Food – Not concoctions with chemical additives.
2. Don't eat anything your great-grandmother wouldn't recognize as food.
3. Avoid food products containing ingredients that no ordinary human would keep in the pantry – What in the world is Ammonium Sulfate??
4. Avoid food products that contain high-fructose corn syrup. These foods are worse for you than sugar.
5. Avoid food products that have some form of sugar (or sweetener) listed among the top three ingredients. Sugar is sugar! Try to avoid it all.
6. Avoid food products with "lite", "low fat" or "nonfat" in their names – almost always very high in sugar.
7. Avoid foods you see advertised on television. Heavily promoted foods are usually processed.
8. Buy your snacks at the farmers market or a healthy market. Fresh dried fruits & nuts.
9. Eat only foods that have been cooked by humans. Not corporations!
10. If it came from a plant, eat it; if it was made IN a plant, don't.
11. Be very careful with starches. They decrease the hormones that make us feel full and increase the hormones that make us feel hungry.
12. No empty calories. Eat nutritionally dense foods.
13. Eat sweet foods as you find them in nature. In nature, sweet foods are packed with fiber. Eat the fruit rather than drink its juice. Don't drink your fruit!
14. The whiter the bread, the sooner you'll be dead.
15. Eat protein at every meal.
16. Do not eat bread for breakfast.
17. Think of processed food as an imposter; not real food.
18. Brown rice only, not white rice – ½ cup only at a sitting
19. Egg whites are great, all protein & only 20 calories. You can eat up to 6 per day.
20. Don't get your fuel from the same place your car does. Do not eat in gas stations. They are processed corn stations! Ethanol outside, high-fructose corn syrup inside.

21. Treat treats as treats, they are special.
22. Break the rules once in a while. All things in moderation, including moderation.
23. Eat normally every day. If you just limit yourself to yogurt, fruit and vegetables you are 50 times more likely to splurge and overeat when you go out.
24. Eating early is key for keeping energy & metabolism up and for weight control. Eat dinner between 5 & 6 pm.
25. Over-indulged? Make the next day all protein.
26. You get maximum pleasure from a food at the third and fourth bite. So take smaller portions or put the fork down early. You will not recapture the pleasure of these earlier bites. Don't eat that tenth spoonful of ice cream.
27. Eat slowly. No "Hovering".

Cooking Tips

28. Use sea salt. It's healthy; it brings the flavor out in foods. If you don't like salt, add a dash of vinegar. It heightens flavors. Stock a good red wine vinegar and a good balsamic. Lemon zest will do the same.
29. Use red pepper of chilies. They speed up your metabolism.
30. Use fresh herbs whenever you can. Favorites to use are fresh are basil, cilantro and rosemary.
31. Garlic, garlic, garlic! It works its wonders in almost any dish or vegetable. Try sautéed broccoli with garlic oil. Delectable! Don't have fresh? Dehydrated flakes are also great.
32. Play with spices. Make any recipe your own signature dish. Buy a few exotic spices and experiment. Throw them in soup, in eggs, even on pizza. Yes, pizza is fine. Get thin crust and load with protein.
33. Find a couple of dishes you like to eat and make them over and over again. You'll find it easier and be much less likely to overeat.
34. Put spaghetti sauce on veggies instead of pasta (think yellow squash, zucchini, brussel sprouts, broccoli). Add cheese and hot pepper flakes. This is low-carb Italian! You'll be surprised at how tasty it is.

35. Only eat treats you make yourself (like French fries, cake or pie). It won't be that often and will taste vastly better.
36. Keep it crunchy. Do not overcook your vegetables. We were designed to chew. It releases enzymes key to digestion.
37. Eat lots of spinach. It is 43% protein AND raises metabolism. Try sautéing in olive oil with garlic, sea salt and lemon pepper! Toss any leftovers in broth for a nice soup. Remember Popeye was "strong to the finish!"
38. If you have cravings, stall for 15 minutes and the cravings will pass. Or eat 6 walnut halves, known to reduce cravings.
39. Try cutting up turnips and parsnips. Spray with oil and cook at 450 degrees for 15 minutes. (Use your favorite spices on top of the oil & toss).
40. Play around with kale. Only 50 calories per bunch!

Eating Out
41. Split entrees. Order something delicious and fun. Get an extra plate (even if you have to pay an extra plate charge of a few dollars). Sit back, relax and enjoy. This allows you to eat delicious food without gaining weight. My husband and I have done this for years. We never feel deprived. Besides, this makes the ordering and eating more interesting.
42. Eat a great hamburger with all the fixings . . . protein-style (tucked into lettuce leaves instead of a bun). I do this once per week.
43. Chefs don't mind if you ask for take away. Really! Don't be hesitant. You now have tomorrow's lunch or breakfast! Just don't take the bread!
44. Whenever you travel, eat like the locals . . . fresh food! No processed foods. Don't eat breakfast in your hotel if it consists of toast or bagels or boxed cereal.
45. It's NOT food if it arrived through the window of your car.

Sugar

46. Don't eat foods that have sweetener in the first 5 ingredients.
47. Control your sugar intake. If you're going to eat a dessert, don't put sugar in your coffee.
48. Eat chocolate. Yes that's right, you heard me. But not chocolate cake or brownies. I mean a really good piece of dark bittersweet chocolate.

- Psychological Trick: The more bars you have around the house the more control you will have over not polishing off the whole bar. Try it! When you see a little stack of bars, it feels less like a "forbidden fruit".
- Also, no chocolate until the end of the day. If you follow this rule for a week or two you will stop craving chocolate at other times.
- Remember, if you're going to eat chocolate, it has to be good chocolate... at least 73% cacao.

49. Experiment with coffee. Find a roast that you love without heavy doses of half & half and sugar. Coffee is good for you!
50. Don't have a "little" sugar if it leads you to have a lot. If you can't just eat a couple of tablespoons of ice cream at a time, don't buy ice cream OR, make yourself walk to the ice cream parlor, get a cone, and walk back! If you don't live near one, park your car far away.
51. Be careful with artificial sweeteners. Your body still thinks it has had sugar and insulin can spike. Stevia is best, but even that can set you off. If you feel hungry after consuming Stevia, that's your clue that it's not for you.

Snacks

52. Never walk and eat. Snacks are not accessories.
53. Feeling hungry before dinner is normal. Don't reach for a snack. Hold off.
54. Craving snacks? Eat more protein at your meals. A handful of walnuts will curb cravings. Or taste something spicy.
55. Eat foods that take time... an artichoke, pistachios in the shell, a tangerine. Give your mind the message that you are eating, and you're stomach will get in sync.

56. Never eat out of a bag.
57. No carb snacks after lunch. They increase cravings and hunger.

Eat What You Love

58. Cut out foods that don't offer pleasure. No knoshing on junk!
59. Become a picky eater . . . a food snob. Want to eat chocolate? Make it the best.
60. At holidays or celebrations only eat your favorite things. Let the rest just be a feast for the eyes.
54. Once in a while, enjoy your favorite treat. No guilt.

You can do it! Call me if you need help!
No More Frankencarbs for You!

"Trust in the LORD with all your heart and lean not on your own understanding; in all your ways acknowledge him, and he will make your paths straight."
Proverbs 3:5-6

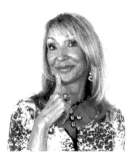

Repeat After Me: "I Am NOT Stuck With This Extra Weight!"

Chapter 10

The Hormone, Brain & Weight Connection

Okay, let's talk about the "muffin top" or "spare tire". You've all seen older people with trim tummies. That can be YOU. Oh, how much younger you will look!

Again, hormones are key!

Metabolism & Hormones: When hormones decline in menopause, metabolism declines about 10-20%. That is why we need to eat differently (higher protein) and/or use the proper supplements.

If not, we accumulate body fat!

The Muffin Top/Spare Tire Syndrome:

You look down at your waist and see a POOCH. Some "pooch" is okay. It is probably God's plan for us to have a little extra weight around the middle as we get older, however... Why do we get that big pooch?

1) Estrogen Dominance: A hormone imbalance that can be corrected by natural progesterone.

2) Insulin Resistance: Your body is not reacting properly to insulin, so your brain is signaled to make more. You makes you constantly hungry AND you store fat.

3) High stress: Numerous cortisol receptor sites exist around the midsection. Adipose tissue has 4 times more receptor sites than the rest of the body! Stress raises cortisol levels, so fat accumulates there when the stress hormones dominate your hormone profile. Progesterone can help counteract this!

Note: Insulin Resistance and High Cortisol are related how? High Cortisol causes a decrease in insulin sensitivity.

Dieting Does Not Work: Seriously!

When you restrict calories, your body adjusts accordingly. Your metabolism slows! If you work on brain chemistry **PLUS** eating habits, you will lose weight because your metabolism will stay strong.

"Will Power" is not the answer! **"Brain Power"** is the answer. Your brain is "command central" when it comes to weight loss. The brain needs certain nutrients and if it does not get those nutrients, it sends out a hunger signal that results in you over-eating.

The Solution: Use Hormones and Nourish Your Brain. This is the way to lose weight AND feel great!

What are the 3 brain chemicals that will help you lose weight?

1. Dopamine – A natural amphetamine, which raises metabolism:
- Dopamine "kick-starts" your metabolism
- Good dopamine levels allow you to experience one helping of a food and then walk away
- Dopamine makes you feel satisfied. Your body gets the message that you are full.
- Dopamine cuts cravings for sugar
- Low dopamine = high cortisol = belly fat

Low dopamine symptoms:
- You need more food than a normal person to feel "satisfied"
- You often wake up tired
- Your energy spikes after eating…so you constantly snack
- You crave simple carbs (Cakes, chips, pasta, pastries, potatoes, white breads & rice)

To increase dopamine naturally
Consume amino acids (specifically phenlyalanine & tyrosine) found in protein rich meats, poultry, fish, & many vegetables, especially:
- Beef (lean cuts), chicken, cottage cheese, eggs, oat flakes, pork
- A single serving of cottage cheese ½ cup greatly increases tyrosine which increases dopamine. Try adding some spices. Personally, I like to add chili powder and turmeric.

Supplements to enhance dopamine:
- L-Tyrosine–stimulates body to burn up adipose tissue, promotes satiety (500 – 1000 mg)
- Folic Acid–increases amount of calories burned (400–800 mg)
- Phosphatidylserine–raises dopamine, lowers cortisol (200 mg)
- Rhodiola rosea –increases sensitivity of neurons to the presence of dopamine (500 mg)
- Vitamin D–controls metabolic syndrome (1000–2000 IU)

2. Serotonin – The "happiness" neurotransmitter. Makes us feel serene, fresh & happy. Helps control cravings!

Low serotonin symptoms:
- You want carbs with every meal
- You crave salty snacks (pickles, olives)
- You crave chocolate
- You get up and eat in the middle of the night
- You have no appetite in the morning
- You consume fewer calories during day, but at night you raid the refrigerator . . . look for high carb snacks
- Panic attacks
- Sad, depressed mood
- You think about food all the time
- Cravings get worse around time of menstrual cycle (in younger women). During the menstrual cycle, body needs more serotonin. You are especially vulnerable to cravings

Causes of Low Serotonin:
- Hormone imbalance (low progesterone)
- Environmental toxins
- Stress (eats up serotonin)
- Lack of sleep
- Lack of sun
- Prescription drugs

Foods That Increase Serotonin Levels:
- Avocado
- chicken
- cottage cheese
- eggs
- yogurt
- turkey

Supplements to enhance serotonin:
- Vitamin D–elevates mood, causes body to burn fat. Take in the morning (2000–4000 IU)
- Melatonin–Suppresses body weight and visceral fat accumulation the day after you take it. Take at night (1.2–9 mg)
- 5-HTP–reduces appetite, promotes weight loss, take at night (50–100 mg)
- DHEA–helps burn belly fat (women:10–20 mg/ Men:10–50 mg)
- SAM-e–can help raise serotonin levels & reduce food cravings (400 mg)

Serotonin-enhancing hormones:
- Progesterone: 40 – 80 mg per day
- Pregnenelone: 50 mg per day. Every other month.

3. GABA (Gamma-Aminobutyric acid) – Promotes calm, stable brain chemistry
- The brain's calming agent
- Helps maintain the proper brain rhythm; keeps brain signals flowing in a calm, steady stream versus shaky "pulses"

- Keeps you feeling balanced (not tense, irritable, hungry)
- Counteracts emotional eating
- Gives control over impulse overeating. You can eliminate the eating you do to control feelings of panic.

Are you GABA deficient?
- You have a second helping at every meal
- You binge at a buffet or you can eat a box of cookies in one sitting
- You eat off someone else's plate mindlessly
- You always order dessert just because it is there

Benefits of taking GABA for weight control:
- Stops stressful eating
- Helps with portion control, over-eating
- Cuts cravings for alcohol/drugs, junk food binges
- Cuts cravings due to anxiety
- Can also help migraines, panic attacks, insomnia

GABA is available as a nutritional supplement. Take 550 mg daily. With GABA you can become one of these people you see eating leisurely and laying down their fork without finishing every morsel on their plate. How wonderful! You are no wonder control!

My favorite product is ZenMind (GABA mixed with L-theanine)

Self-Test
Let's pinpoint your needs for YOUR weight loss success.
Note: You could possibly need more than 1 brain supplement.

Is This You?
1) I need energy. I am consuming excessive amounts of coffee and sugar to get going and keep going during the day. I want to constantly snack because food seems to give me energy.

You need DOPAMINE
Eat more protein
L-Tyrosine is good for you

2) I often crave salty foods. I am not hungry in the morning, but I can eat all night long. I look for high carb snacks. I get up at night to snack. I eat small snacks, but many of them. I have trouble falling asleep at night.

You need SEROTONIN
Eat foods high in tryptophan (the precursor to serotonin)
Use spices in abundance
5-HTP is especially good for you!

3) I binge. I over-eat. I have no portion control. I feel addicted to some foods. When I'm stressed I eat whatever will calm me down. I don't feel like my brain ever tells me to stop eating. I am an emotional eater.

You need GABA
Drink green tea (2-4 cups) for calmness, attention, & focus.
Decrease caffeine, eat only complex carbs & high fiber foods.
Zen Mind is great for you!

In summary, here is what you may need:
1. **Dopamine:** for energy & metabolism
2. **Serotonin:** for a calm & restful brain and to eliminate cravings for carbs & salty foods
3. **GABA:** for obsessive/anxious eating patterns & to help you develop portion control

WEIGHT LOSS & SLEEP
You must sleep correctly to help you lose weight

FACT: The more tired you are, the heavier you will get. Sleep influences the hormone that regulates satiety and hunger. Leptin levels fall when you are sleep deprived.

Also…**growth hormone declines with sleep deprivation.** One week of poor sleep inhibits growth hormone. HGH controls the body's proportion of muscle & fat so low levels lead to weight gain.

IMPORTANT:
- You need 7-8 hours of restful sleep.
- You need a 90 min cycle to reach <u>restorative</u> phase: this phase promotes release of neuro-chemicals.
- Proper sleep resets hormones.
- Sleep helps increase metabolism
- Sleep lowers cortisol levels – discourages belly fat accumulation and insulin resistance

<u>Conclusion</u>

Weight loss is not about "will power." If it was, all of you magnificent women and men who are out there and those who call my office every day would not be struggling with this problem.

Your brain chemistry & hormones need to be optimized so that your body will have a natural ability to:
- **Eliminate cravings**
- **Control your appetite**
- **Stay motivated (because you feel good)**
- **Have a calm, happy, and balanced mood**
- **Eliminate feelings of stress and deprivation**

This strategy really works! Please let me know of your progress. Call me if you have questions as you are going along. I want to help you!

"More than that, we rejoice in our sufferings, knowing that suffering produces endurance, and endurance produces character, and character produces hope, and hope does not put us to shame, because God's love has been poured into our hearts through the Holy Spirit who has been given to us."
Romans 5:3-5

Chapter 11

Calling All Girls!
Unwanted Facial Hair

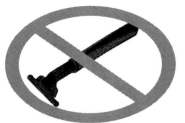

Yikes! For women this is definitely aging, not to mention distressing. I want you to have a smooth, beautiful face. If I can do it, you can too!

Since I began talking to women about their hormones, there has been a huge increase in this complaint. It is happening to younger and younger women – even teenagers.
There are several factors that cause facial hair. Let's take a look.

Excessive growth of facial and body hair can be indicative of hormonal imbalance between estrogen-testosterone-progesterone. Progesterone acts as a regulator for the entire endocrine system and is needed to achieve the proper balance between these hormones. As you have learned, many women are deficient in this vital hormone.

Facial hair growth can also be related to diet (highly processed foods and excess sugar are big culprits). Women who are constantly exposed to the effects of a poor diet, high stress levels, and xenoestrogens in addition to being deficient in progesterone can see unwanted hair growth.

Also, as women age and their ovarian function slows down, they can produce more androgens (male hormones) causing an increase in facial hair.

I believe that progesterone is the first line of defense (natural, NOT synthetic). Both menopausal and menstruating women report facial hair decreases or disappears after 4 – 6 months of progesterone use. They used the cream consistently and applied it twice per day. They often rubbed some of the progesterone directly on the hair.

This process takes patience! In about 3 months you should see the facial hairs starting to thin out. In 6 months they will become less coarse and less dark. The tip of the chin is usually the last place to go. You can just keep plucking those until they disappear. Plucking does not exacerbate the hair growth.

Some women have hirsutism due to adrenal malfunction and may need some adrenal support supplements, so I also suggest use of adrenal nourishment (see chapter 3). You could begin with progesterone alone OR, if budget permits, use both progesterone and an adrenal supplement simultaneously. Don't worry. This is totally reversible!

By the way there is a process offered in dermatologist and Plastic surgeon offices called "dermaplaning". The technician will take a thin razor blade and literally will "shave off" some of those fine white hairs that grow on the side of your face. I've had it done to the fine tune of $175 and all it is fine hair shaving. You can do it yourself before a night out or important event. The hair does not grow back thicker.

"You are altogether beautiful, my love; there is no flaw in you."
Song of Solomon 4:7

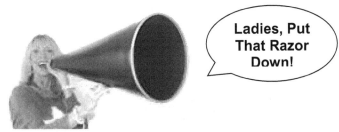

Ladies, Put That Razor Down!

Chapter 12

Detox That Beautiful Body & Prolong Your Life

Did you know there are estrogens in the environment?
Yes . . . lots of them depending on where you live.
These are extraneous estrogens that are affecting our bodies and causing us to have hormone imbalance. When our body is overloaded with toxins skin gets dull, and we feel sluggish.
What is our worst toxin? **Xenoestrogens!**
For a younger you, banish those xenoestrogens from your life!

What are Xenoestrogens?
Xeno means foreign, so xenoestrogens are "foreign" estrogens; that is, made from something outside the body. Many are petrochemically-based or are by-products of petrochemical production. These substances have an estrogenic effect when they enter the human body. Birth control pills are also foreign or "chemical estrogens"

How do Xenoestrogens disrupt hormone balance?
These nasty synthetic chemicals bind directly to hormone receptor sites in our body, activating the sites and blocking our normal hormone activity. They accumulate in the tissues and wreak havoc on our ability to metabolize and eliminate toxins, in addition to creating a state of excess estrogen in the body.

The disturbing effects for men and women:
- A 50% decrease in sperm count since 1938
- An increased incidence of testicular & prostate cancer
- A potentiating or stimulating effect in breast cancer
- A potentiating or stimulating effect in endometriosis
- Endometrial cancer
- Premenstrual syndrome (PMS)
- Fibrocystic Breast Syndrome
- Postmenopausal osteoporosis

Sources of Xenoestrogens

- Paints & Textiles
- Paper products
- Solvents and adhesives
- Pesticide residue on fruits & vegetables
- Herbicides– used on lawns & plants
- Car exhaust
- Nearly all plastics, plastic wraps (leak into food)
- Industrial waste (PCBs) & dioxins
- Livestock fed estrogenic drugs to fatten them.
- Tobacco smoke
- Some city water supplies
- Some commercial household cleaning supplies
- Insect repellants

Look for these ingredients and try to purchase products that do NOT contain them:

- Dioxins
- PCB's (Polychlorinated biphenyls)
- Bisphenol A
- Phthalates

Do-It-Yourself Protection

- Whenever possible, purchase organically grown fruits and vegetables. I know it can be expensive, but at least try to do it with anything you use in abundance. I eat organic lettuce because I eat lettuce daily. Highest pesticide foods include: strawberries, peaches, bell peppers, apples, green beans. Wash these thoroughly.
- Buy meat and dairy products that are hormone-free.
- Don't eat fat on meat/poultry - chemicals collect there.
- Do not purchase food/drink packaged in plastic wrap or styrofoam containers.
- Remove plastic wraps as soon as you get home, because the longer the plastic is in contact with food, the more the xenoestrogens may leach into the food. Store food in butcher paper, wax paper, freezer paper, foil or glass when possible. Use glass or ceramic storage containers.

- Never microwave food in plastic or Styrofoam containers. Use a glass or ceramic dish instead. When plastic is heated, it diffuses rapidly into food. If you need a lid, use a flat dish or a piece of freezer paper or damp paper towel.

A Dartmouth University study showed that plastic wrap heated in a microwave in vegetable oil had 500,000 times the minimum amount of xenoestrogens needed to stimulate breast cancer cells to grow.

- Invest in a water filter or drink bottle water. In some areas, xenoestrogens are prevalent in drinking water due to massive amounts of detergents used by industries that make their way to ground water.
- Avoid baby formula sold in polycarbonate (clear plastic) bottles. If possible, use only glass baby bottles. If you use polycarbonate bottles, don't heat/microwave them.
- Use organic pesticides. Unless it's an emergency. Avoid having your home sprayed with chemicals by an exterminator. If so, stay away from the house for 8 hours.
- Avoid herbicides. Instead, use a cup of salt in a gallon of vinegar.
- Replace chemical-based household cleaning products with natural products.
- Do not give plastic toys to babies or toddlers who will put them in their mouths.
- Avoid solvents

Without these xenoestrogens you are on your way to Better Health and a more Beautiful body!

"He saved us, not because of works done by us in righteousness, but according to his own mercy, by the washing of regeneration and renewal of the Holy Spirit,"
Titus 3:5

Chapter 13

Calling All Men

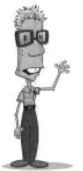

> **Will work for testosterone!**

Hello fellas!

Are you over the age of 40? Not feeling as peppy, vigorous and robust as you used to?

Do you have any of these symptoms of hormone imbalance? (Known as "Andropause")

- Burned out feeling
- Weight gain
- Abdominal fat or "spare tire"
- Decreased mental clarity
- Decreased sex drive
- Increased urinary urge
- Decreased strength & stamina
- Superficial or nervous sleep
- Irritable / anxious
- Depressed / lack of inner peace
- Bloated
- Night sweats
- Muscle tension (especially shoulders & neck)
- Poor concentration
- Sluggish / lethargic
- Erectile Dysfunction
- Unable to lose weight
- Male pattern baldness
- Prostate problems

If so, your answer could be as simple as the use of a bio-identical progesterone cream.

Experts agree that progesterone can help:
- Prostate problems / prostate health
- Energy & libido
- Excess weight around the mid-section
- "Breast" development
- Overall sense of well-being
- Hair health / male pattern baldness
- Anyone using a statin drug (which decreases progesterone)
- Prevent coronary artery disease

You say:
"Barbara, why would a man need supplemental progesterone? Isn't that a female hormone?"
No, progesterone is unisex; made in both the male and female body. Men produce progesterone in smaller amounts that women do, but it is still vital.
Progesterone is the primary precursor to a man's sex hormones, specifically testosterone. A man's progesterone is produced in his adrenal glands and his testes.

Here is why you may be low in this important "Feel Good" hormone.
1. **As a male ages, his progesterone level decreases** just as it does in women. In men, this occurs around age 45.
    a) When a man's progesterone levels decrease, his 5-alpha reductase enzyme converts his "good" testosterone to di-hydro testosterone, a form of testosterone which stimulates the prostate. The prostate gland will swell and enlarge. Progesterone is a potent inhibitor of 5-alpha-reductase. Many of you have heard of the drug finasteride (Proscar). Proscar inhibits the enzyme 5-alpha reductase, but progesterone can do just as good a job and is NATURAL.
    b) Progesterone deficiency exposes a man to other diseases associated with excess estrogen such as ischemic heart disease and male pattern baldness.

2. **Xenoestrogens (from the environment) negatively affect men just as they do women.** Estrogen dominance caused by xenoestrogens is affecting men by raising their estrogen levels to dangerous levels. Men naturally make estrogen and estradiol, but in much lower amounts than women. Xenoestrogens cause the estrogen levels in men to rise. Testosterone is a direct antagonist of estradiol (an estrogen). When testosterone levels fall and the shift from testosterone to DHT occurs, the effect of estradiol (estrogen) increases. Men developing "breasts" can often be a sign of this estrogen effect. Also, lack of energy, decreased interest in life, and a "poochy" tummy can be signs of elevated estrogen in men. Dr. Francisco Contreras, founder of The Oasis of Hope Cancer Center, calls this "biochemical chaos". He advises that progesterone balances the negative effects of these environmental estrogens.

3. **Estrogen Dominance in General.** In men, estrogen gradually rises with age. Estrogen levels especially increase in aging men who are overweight because fat cells manufacture estrogens. The more fat a man carries on his body, the higher his estradiol levels will be. Thus, with aging and weight gain, estrogen dominance occurs. Even if a man's testosterone levels are normal, if his estradiol levels are high, he can have estrogen dominance. The symptoms are **larger than normal breasts, anxiety, insomnia, prostate enlargement, weight gain, and gall bladder problems.**

4. **Testosterone Deficiency.** According to Thierry Hertoghe, M.D, a leading expert in hormone therapy, progesterone can block   5-alpha reductase and increase testosterone.

How Does Progesterone Protect Against Prostate Cancer?
Research shows that the prostate is embryologically similar to the female uterus. Hence it is subject to the negative influences of estrogen dominance in the same way as a woman's breast and uterus is. Natural progesterone balances or opposes excess estrogen. Progesterone prevents a man's

body from converting his "good" testosterone to di-hydro testosterone. Thus, a man's testosterone remains in the "good" form—for virility, energy, libido, and weight control. "Good" Testosterone does NOT cause prostate cancer. Think about it . . . if this were true 19 and 20 year-old males would be developing prostate cancer as these are the individuals with the highest levels.

Research of John R. Lee, M.D., and Other Experts
Testosterone Levels: Progesterone, like finasteride and saw palmetto, stops the conversion of testosterone to DHT. In this manner, progesterone helps raise testosterone levels. **Testosterone remains Testosterone.**

Weight Loss: Progesterone, like testosterone, is an anabolic hormone, meaning that it helps burn fat for energy. Thus, it helps keep men from becoming obese. With less body fat, there is less endogenous (within the body) estrone production. Take back your waist line!
It will be fun and you will feel trim, fit & fabulous. I guarantee it!

Cancer Prevention: Dr. Lee used progesterone for over 30 years in his practice. He had a large number of anecdotal stories of complete reversals of metastatic prostatic cancers. The clinical research is on-going. There is strong biochemical evidence to support this recommendation.

All cells, with the exception of brain and muscle cells, multiply continuously. The genes which regulate this cell growth are p53 and bcl2. If the gene bcl2 dominates it will push cells to cancer. If gene p53 dominates the opposite will occur and the cell growth is controlled and the cancer does not occur.

Both progesterone and testosterone **turn on the anti-cancer gene p53!** Estradiol (estrogen), on the other hand, stimulates Bcl 2 production, which increases the risk of cancer. According to Dr. Lee, men using natural progesterone have protection against prostate cancer. Dr. Francisco Contreras also says all men should use progesterone, especially those who feel like "half the man I used to be." Is that you?

Hair Loss: DHT generates male pattern baldness. Progesterone reduces DHT levels.

Anxiety: Progesterone calms the central nervous system. This is especially helpful to men who are tense or anxious.

Interested in Fertility?

Estrogen dominance and xenoestrogens such as those found in pesticides & insecticides (Xenoestrogens) can decrease the sperm count in men causing infertility.
Since the introduction of pesticides and the wide development of certain plastics, the sperm count in men has dropped over the past few decades. A majority of pesticides have estrogenic effects and excess estrogen can reduce male fertility.

According to John R. Lee, Dr. Thierry Hertoghe, and other leading experts, **natural progesterone blocks the estrogens and sperm count returns to normal.**
Progesterone also stimulates sperm motility. Studies exist that have shown the direct link between pesticides and infertility in men – a study in the Netherlands published in The Lancet makes this direct link and provides significant data.

The study showed a strong correlation between poor sperm quality in men and the use of pesticides on the job. The highest-risk jobs: livestock farmers, fruit & flower growers, and gardeners.

It is widely recognized that men are generally more involved with spraying pesticides in the garden or on weeds. They are also more apt to use insecticides, particularly on ants around the home. Please be careful. Many of these common insecticides and pesticides can be absorbed through the skin. Wash carefully after handling any such substances. Wear a mask when using these chemicals OR consider leaving those weeds in your garden.

To Sum It Up, As Men Age

1. Testosterone is converted to dihydrotestosterone (DHT) by 5-alpha-reductase enzyme, stimulating prostate growth.
2. "Good' Testosterone levels fall, DHT rises
3. Progesterone levels fall
4. Estrogen-effect increases (both bodily produced and environmental)

Progesterone Dosage For Men

The dose of natural progesterone for men is 10 to 12 mg per day. Men do NOT need time off like women and can take the progesterone continuously. When using ProMEN, use ¼ tsp once daily. If using ProHELP, use 1/8 tsp. once a day.

Both ProHELP and ProMEN contain USP progesterone which is an exact match, that is, bio-identical, to human progesterone.

Natural progesterone may counteract both the conversion of testosterone to DHT as well as oppose the estrogen effect, restoring a man to BALANCE.

Where / When Do Men Apply Progesterone?

Areas of application should be where the capillaries are abundant; the back of the hand, palm of the hand or inner arm or wrist. It may also be applied directly to the perineum. The best time to apply progesterone is about ½ hour to 1 hour before bedtime.

Should I Use Progesterone?

Dr. Lee and other leading experts have stated that nearly all men should seriously consider **natural progesterone replacement** sometime in their 40s, or even earlier if they have a family history of prostate cancer. They believe that progesterone can lower the risk of prostate cancer.

I have heard back from hundreds of men or their wives who report:

- **Prostate problems have disappeared**
- **Energy has increased**
- **Libido has increased**
- **Hair has regrown (It has also been reported that the use of progesterone has a reasonable likelihood of decreasing male balding).**
- **Stomach fat has disappeared**
- **Depression has disappeared**
- **Insomnia has ceased**

Personally, I do not have <u>any</u> reports from any men who said their doctors recommended they not use progesterone. Results of less muscle tension & anxiety & better sleep may be immediate. Maximum effects are felt in 4-6 weeks.

Testimonials of Progesterone:

"I had every symptom of prostate enlargement and also had no true energy or libido. My wife bought me a jar of ProMEN and I had almost immediate relief. My symptoms have disappeared and I am "feeling my oats" again, if you know what I mean. I want to tell you, men, this product has changed me back into the man I used to be!
J. A., Seattle, WA

"I am a 73 year old man. I was really dragging all the time; constantly fatigued. I have to work 8 hours per day and I was always tired. My wife heard about ProMEN and ordered it for me. I have used 2 jars and my fatigue is gone! I feel like a brand new man!" **J.T., Houston, TX**

"In my career I experience a lot of stress. I experienced years of insomnia from stress. I would only sleep an hour or two and wake up every night. When I learned about the progesterone crème, I knew that was a very important key. The first night I used the ProMEN, I slept like a baby. Using the crème every day, I noticed a definite boost in energy throughout the day. Also, my prostate has returned to the size it was before I was 50." **M.S., Dallas, TX**

Progesterone can help YOU be a "Younger You."
Now, that's a good thing!

"He is like a tree planted by streams of water that yields its fruit
in its season, and its leaf does not wither.
In all that he does, he prospers."
Psalm 1:1-4

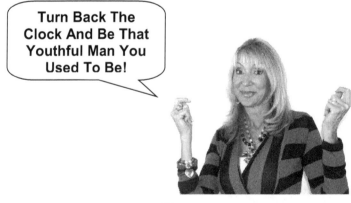

Chapter 14

Sweet Sleep, Sweet Dreams

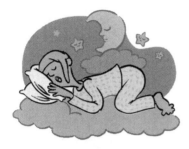

"Sweet Sleep" is paramount to our Younger You, Younger Me program!
Are you one of those people who no longer can get a good night's sleep? Are you waking up at 2 or 3 in the morning; lying in bed tossing and turning? Are you desperate for just one good long peaceful sleep?

I can help!
Sleep is seriously important! When people don't sleep for 3 days in a row, they can become psychotic! As a matter of fact, sleep deprivation has been used as a form of torture. Many of you can relate to that feeling of desperation when you cannot sleep.
Don't accept insomnia as part of growing old!
Good sleep increases longevity and contributes to feeling hale and robust.

The Problem with insomnia
If you do not get your proper sleep, your hormones will suffer!
A disturbance in your circadian rhythm can result in hormone deficiencies and imbalances.

In addition, lack of sleep has an aging effect on the body. Sleep-deprived people look burdened, weak and worst of all become irritable and grouchy. Now that's NOT youthful.

Is this you?

- You experience poor sleep: a superficial or anxious sleep
- You wake easily during the night
- It is difficult for you to fall asleep, fall back asleep, or both
- You rarely dream
- Restless legs at night
- Tense muscles at night
- Fatigue during the day, and even upon arising
- Eyes look tired, bags under eyes
- Poor skin tone, wrinkles and furrows
- Anxiety, lack of inner peace, especially at night
- Excessive emotions, irritability
- Early graying of hair
- Flabby muscles

So, sound like you? Melatonin, "the sleep hormone" can help.

If you cannot sleep, you are not deficient in Ambien, Lunesta, or other popular sleep drugs. It is melatonin deficiency that causes insomnia.
Melatonin is not a sleeping pill. It is a hormone. It will reset your circadian rhythm back to normal. It can take from 1 week to six weeks to accomplish this.
A sleeping pill does NOT restore normal sleep cycles, so when you discontinue them, insomnia returns.

My Story

I had quite a few of these symptoms and once I started taking supplemental melatonin, they disappeared within 3 weeks. Also, my dear husband, a chronic insomniac is now sleeping like the proverbial baby. He does not even wake up when the dog is whining to go out! Maybe I need to hide his melatonin. Just kidding. Before I got him on it, the poor man was not able to sleep through the night for almost 2 years straight. Now he is so well rested, it has actually helped him with his weight. Did you know that good sleep lowers cortisol levels (the stress hormone)? High cortisol leads to weight gain right around the middle. You know the infamous "Spare Tire" that no one wants to see on themselves or their loved one. So, you really can sleep yourself slender.

Directions for Melatonin Use

- Take melatonin about 45 minutes to 1 hour before you plan to sleep. Begin with a dose of about 3 milligrams
- You can take additional melatonin if you repeatedly wake up during the night, using the supplement to create deeper sleep. However, give it a try for a week or so before moving on to a higher dose
- Use melatonin to reset your body clock when you experience jet lag by taking it at the appropriate time to sleep in your time zone, even if you are not tired yet
- Watch for any side effects the next day. If you feel groggy, you can take the melatonin earlier in the evening
- Expect some vivid dreams the first week. This is a good thing – a sign you are in deep sleep.

I really like sublingual melatonin that you take about 30 minutes before bedtime.
However, I have another favorite application . . . Topical!
That's right, you just rub it on your face.
And guess what? The restorative power of sleep rejuvenates and repairs the skin, even as the melatonin crème makes the skin softer & more youthful looking. The product I like is called Restful Night. Each ¼ tsp contains 1.2 mg of melatonin.

Other good news: There are no absolute contradictions to taking melatonin unless you have a disease that makes your cortisol needs higher than normal which is very rare. Also, avoid high doses of melatonin during pregnancy. Check with your doctor on this.

What are people saying after they use Melatonin or progesterone crème?
"I started sleeping better right away."
"I sleep so well, I can't even hear my hubby snoring anymore."
"I'm falling asleep like a little baby when I lay my head down."
"It's like a miracle."
"I'm not lying awake for hours feeling anxious and alone."
"Even when I get up to use the bathroom, I fall right back to sleep."

Insomnia from Estrogen Dominance: What can you do?
Estrogen dominance can cause severe insomnia. Estrogen is a central nervous system stimulant. Progesterone, on the other hand has a calming effect on the brain.

A majority of women experience relief from insomnia when they begin using natural progesterone. Women reported excellent results when they rubbed their evening dose on the back of their neck, sometimes using a slightly larger dose in the evening. Remember, progesterone has a calming effect on the central nervous system and it also balances out the excess estrogens that can be exciting the brain. Hormonal balance promotes good, healthy sleep.

Other Sleep Tips!
1. Calcium has been known to promote sleep by its calming effect on the nervous system. Take the largest portion of your daily calcium supplement at bedtime, OR eat a high calcium snack.

2. Eliminate caffeinated beverages after 12 noon. Did you know that it takes caffeine between 6-8 hours to be cleared from your body?

3. Drink tea. Alternate some herbal teas that you like. Good options are lemon, elderberry, chamomile and licorice. You can also find teas called "Sleepy Time" or "Nighty Night" which contain sleep-promoting herbs.

4. Do any physical activity in the late afternoon or early evening. Your muscles need to be tired. The best sleep occurs when the body is cool, so take hot baths 1-2 hours before bedtime, not immediately before retiring.

5. Melatonin, the sleep hormone, is extremely sensitive to light and will "scatter" when exposed to light. Live a "melatonin-friendly" lifestyle. Keep your bedroom dark. Use a digital clock with low light or turn it toward the wall. If you get up to go to the bathroom at night, use

only a dim night light. Do not flip on a light switch and flood your brain with light.

6. Avoid alcohol at bedtime. Even though it may make you feel drowsy, alcohol interferes with the brains sleep mechanisms and you will not have a restful night's sleep.

7. Try relaxation exercises before going to sleep. A great exercise is to take 10 deep breaths, wait 5 minutes and take 10 more. Repeat several times. Deep breathing works wonders, even if you wake up in the night.

8. Lavender oil placed on your pillow can help promote sleep. Put it on a cotton swab and place on or near the pillow.

9. If you get up frequently in the night to use the bathroom, have your last beverage with dinner.

10. Avoid looking at the clock. This can promote more anxiety and lead to more difficulty falling asleep. Face the clock to the wall.

11. Do not watch television in bed just before turning out your light. This is a habit for so many people, but it is the worst thing you can do. First, it is very stimulating to the brain and secondly, it does not promote the idea that your bed is for sleeping. Reading is fine – calm and restful.

12. If you do wake up in the middle of the night, do not do anything stimulating. Some women have told me that they just start reading the dictionary!

13. Eat "sleepytime snacks" at night. These include bananas, celery and celery juice, wheat germ, brown rice, warm milk, lemon water with honey.

14. Figs – Seriously! Women have told me that when they ate figs, they slept better, but they did not know why. I did some research and found that figs contain melatonin! If you like figs, try eating 2-3 at night. It works and I include figs as my after-dinner snack.

15. Still can't sleep? Count your blessings. Start with the letter A and add a correlating blessing. Then move on to B. you probably won't make it to Z. studies show that people who are grateful sleep longer and better than people who are less appreciative

A Good Tip: Figure out what time you want to arise in the morning, count back 7-8 hours. Then, set your alarm for when you want to go to sleep INSTEAD of when you want to wake up.

Important
If you go to a doctor who prescribes sleeping pills for you, there is important information you should know. They are addictive and can cause severe side effects. In March, 2007 the FDA has recommended adding warnings to 13 separate sleeping pills because of sleep-related behaviors that included sleep-driving, sleep-cooking, severe allergic reactions and severe facial swelling in some women. Also, a side effect of some sleeping pills can actually be insomnia!

Okay. . . This is your assignment: GET YOUR SLEEP!
If you cannot sleep after trying melatonin or progesterone crème or both, CALL ME! I won't give up on you!

I leave you with these verses from the Bible:

For so He gives his beloved sleep
Psalm 127:2

. . . You will lie down and your sleep will be sweet
Psalm 3:24

In other words, we were designed to have a good night's sleep. So, sleep well, my friends.

Chapter 15

Ladies: Lubricate, Lubricate, Lubricate

It's time to talk about vaginal dryness.

One lady called me & explained that she had a very dry "Virginia" You don't want that! It makes most women very cranky and unhappy. Not to mention the negative effects on a marriage. Remember that old adage "When mama's not happy, nobody's happy." And when women are not happy they look older. Let's nourish the "Virginia".

What Has Happened?

Vaginal dryness, vaginal thinning, and what is called "atrophy" are very common problems for menopausal women.

When estrogen levels decline, the vulva loses its collagen, fat and water retaining abilities. As a result, it becomes flattened, thin, dry, and loses tone. Lack of vaginal lubrication also means hormone levels are dropping. Classic symptoms of vaginal atrophy are dryness, irritation, burning, and a feeling of pressure. The vagina gets progressively shorter and narrower and its tissue thins. The vagina also becomes susceptible to infection because the thin walls lack the normal secretions that normally cleanse vaginal tissues. The vaginal pH rises and it becomes more alkaline. This allows undesirable bacteria to replace friendly bacteria. This can result in urinary tract infections.

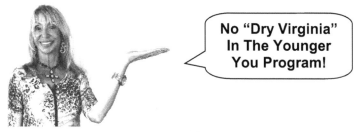

No "Dry Virginia"
In The Younger
You Program!

ALSO, when the body is deficient in progesterone, the estrogen receptors become less sensitive to estrogen. Therefore, even a woman with sufficient estrogen can have vaginal dryness. When progesterone levels are restored in these cases, estrogen receptors become more sensitive and vaginal lubrication returns.

What Can Be Done?

- A 3 month trial of progesterone is found to help many women eliminate vaginal dryness. This is especially helpful news to women with a history of breast cancer who cannot take any form of estrogen. If, after 3 months, you still experience the dryness, and you have lots of hot flashes & night sweats, you may need to add some estrogen.
- If you are no longer having periods, a cream with natural progesterone and containing red clover extract (a phyto-estrogen) has helped many women. A study done in Australia linked an oral supplement containing Red Clover with relief from vaginal dryness. (I believe that the crème form is better absorbed and utilized by the body).
- For women with severe vaginal dryness or who want more immediate relief, there is a wonderful product called Ostaderm V which is a plant based estrogen-progesterone crème that is applied to the vulva area. It contains estriol and I have seen it restore vaginal tissue health very rapidly. Its creator, David Shefrin, N.D. says: "It amazes me how easily the vaginal problems can be reversed." He goes on to say if the atrophy is profound, it may take a few months.
- Vitamin E – Another natural product that studies show to be effective in relieving atrophic vaginitis is Vitamin E. You can pierce the capsule with a pin and insert into the vagina.
- Lubrication – For over-the-counter use, there is a product called Replens that is long-lasting; a single application lasts up to 72 hours. Studies show it can increase vaginal secretions.

If you need more help with this delicate tissue, please email or call. No more "dry Virginia" in your Younger You program!

"Let thy heart cheer thee in the days of thy youth"
Ecclesiastes 11:9

Chapter 16

Supplements For The Younger You

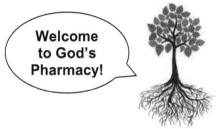

Welcome to God's Pharmacy!

Barbara, you ask, do I really need to take supplements? Do they actually work?

Personally, I am a big supplement taker. Since I began taking supplements 15 years ago I truly feel like a "new" Barbara. Because I have a researcher's heart, I have periodically discontinued my supplement regimen to see if I felt any difference. I tell you friends, within 2 – 3 days I lost that feeling of energetic youthfulness. . . like I could "slay a dragon!" If you want to call me, I can tell you my favorites.

Dr. Mark Hyman, functional medicine specialist writes that only these people do not need supplements: Those who
- Eat wild, fresh, organic, local, non-genetically modified food grown in virgin mineral & nutrient-rich soils that has not been transported across vast distances or stored for months before being eaten
- Work and live outside
- Breath only fresh unpolluted air
- Drink only pure, clean water
- Sleep 9 hours a night
- Move their bodies every day
- Are free from chronic stress & exposure to environmental toxins

I believe this would only be Adam & Eve!
Certainly not us!

I believe supplements are an absolute necessity. They can definitely help you avoid doctor's visits and restore your youthful vitality.

According to a survey of 1,200 doctors, 79% of physicians recommended natural supplements, 72% of those physicians were taking natural supplements for their own health.

You can easily customize your supplement program
You don't need a lot... just what will work for YOU!
It can be VERY inexpensive & make you feel like a new person

Are Supplements Safe?

The U.S. National Poison Data Systems 2009 Annual Report announced that there were ZERO deaths from vitamin supplements, herbal products, homeopathic supplements and over-the-counter hormone products in that year.
Yet over 100,000 patients (in hospitals) died from drugs that they took "appropriately".

This is the difference between
God's Pharmacy and Man's Pharmacy!

My Experience

I started using supplements when I was 34 years old. I was seeing people that seemed to have UNLIMITED energy and vitality. I saw people in their 70's and even 80's who had awesome intellectual focus, memory and youthful vigor. They were impressive in their robust health. Well I said to myself, I want to be like them! So I began a supplement regimen. I take specific supplements for specific needs and I usually take a break on Sunday about twice a month.

Recently, I decided to experiment and took 4 days off from ANY supplements including hormones.
By the 5th day, which was a Sunday, I was DRAGGING! I mean it.... my husband wanted to go to a movie and I was feeling so blah I didn't even want to get in the car.

Recently, a Time Magazine writer wrote about his experience and he said the same thing. After he quit, he said "I don't wake up now with that feeling of the lion who can eat the world". Now I have to tell you, I am almost a senior citizen so without my supplements, I believe I would fall into the category of an "old person". Old persons EXPECT to feel less energetic, sleep less, lose hair, etc. So they often do not question these feelings. I am encouraging you.... you DO NOT need to feel old. I have more energy now and feel better than I did back at 34 years of age.

OKAY... Now let's talk about you!
You don't have to go overboard and take astronomical amounts of supplements.
I am going to take specific categories and tell you what supplements work the best for that need. The suggested doses are in bold type.

I will indicate if a certain supplement is a brand name that may be my favorite product, but I tried to list the ingredients so you could look for a similar product in a health food store.

Energy

DHEA
Also fantastic for memory. See Chapter 2.

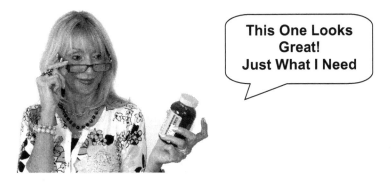

This One Looks Great! Just What I Need

Rhodiola Rosea
For stress relief, stamina, memory.

Rhodiola Rosea is a powerful adaptogenic herb, meaning it "adapts" in your body to give you what you need. It is known for its beneficial effects on energy production and reduction of fatigue.
Though there are more than 20 species of the rhodiola herb, only Rhodiola Rosea contains the 3 active rosavin compounds: Rosavin, Rosin, and Rosarin.

Research
In a 2009 study, researchers found that Rhodiola reduced stress and increased mental performance in adults suffering from fatigue. Rhodiola was also found to reduce fatigue in 56 physicians on night duty in a study published in Phytomedicine. It can also minimize both depression and anxiety.

- Reduces fatigue & increases work capacity
- Improves ability to handle stress
- Enhances mental alertness & improves memory
- Improves capacity for exercise, strength & endurance
- Strengthens nervous system, improving fibromyalgia
- Aids weight reduction
- Increases sexual function
- Stimulates serotonin to help reduce depression
- Improves blood circulation
- A powerful weapon against anxiety

How Does It Work?
Rhodiola is great for increasing energy levels if they're low, and enhancing mental and physical performance. Rather than over-stimulating the adrenals, adaptogens like Rhodiola actually support proper function and help the adrenals produce cortisol in natural patterns.

Instructions: Take 1, 500 mg capsule daily with a meal.

Depression

SAM-e

Also for osteoarthritis, fibromyalgia, and liver disease.
Can work within hours

- **Mood:** Helps you regain control of your good mood. You have brighter days and feel revitalized. Can also raise serotonin levels.
- **Osteoarthritis:** A number of double-blind studies confirm that SAM-e can help individuals with osteoarthritis. SAM-e reduced stiffness, pain and swelling in arthritic joints, as well as improved overall joint health. Scientists have found SAM-e is as effective as ibuprofen and naproxen for arthritis.
- **Fibromyalgia:** Double-blind research suggests that SAM-e can assist those with fibromyalgia. People with fibromyalgia given SAM-e showed a decrease in fatigue, pain sensation, and stiffness. Study participants also noted a significant improvement in mood.
- **Depression:** SAM-e is shown to be more effective for relieving depression than many common anti-depressants. SAM-e does not require a doctor's prescription. In Europe, SAM-e is used like a prescription drug for treating depression. Given SAM-e's impressive safety record, scientists believe that virtually anyone suffering from depression should try it.
- **Food Cravings:** SAM-e crosses the blood – brain barrier and positively affects neurotransmitters. Can help eliminate cravings
- **Liver Cirrhosis:** A wealth of studies show that SAM-e is helpful for various liver conditions including cirrhosis. In one trial, people with liver cirrhosis caused by alcoholism who took SAM-e for two years experienced a nearly 50 lower death rate and/or liver transplantation rate, compared with study participant who received a placebo. It is also helpful for fatty liver disease. Scientists believe SAM-e can prevent the onset and progression of liver disease.
- **Heart:** Can lower levels of homocysteine, an amino acid associated with cardiovascular disease.

Obviously, this is a great supplement for us over age of 50!

5-HTP

Also for Insomnia, & Weight Loss

5-HTP (5-hydroxytryptophan) is a metabolite of the amino acid tryptophan. Tryptophan is broken down by vitamins, enzymes, and other co-factors into 5-HTP, and 5-HTP is then turned into serotonin. Users notice results in as little as 1 day!

5-HTP:
- Stops carbohydrate cravings
- Enhances serotonin, your "feel good" hormone
- Improves mild depression
- Aids restful sleep
- Helps prevent anxiety
- Provides fibromyalgia relief
- Reduces panic attacks
- Aids WEIGHT LOSS

Serotonin is the neurotransmitter that tells your brain that you are satisfied and do not need to eat more. Serotonin deficiency contributes to weight gain, depression, sleeplessness, anxiety, inflammation, and joint pain. Low serotonin also leads to sugar cravings and overeating. 5-HTP *reduces appetite while it enhances your mood, and increases your energy levels.*

A well-controlled trial with obese individuals found a significant weight loss with 5-HTP.
5-HTP has also been extensively researched for the treatment of *depression and anxiety.* 5-HTP's natural relief for depression and related problems also comes without the side effects of pharmaceutical alternatives.

NOTE: 5-HTP is very safe, but if you are taking MAO inhibitors, SSRIs (Prozac, Luvox, Paxil, Effexor, Zoloft) and/or the tricyclic anti-depressants (Elavil, Tofranil, Pamelor), do not take 5-HTP without discussing it with your healthcare provider. 5-HTP is often used to help wean people off of SSRIs and other anti-depressants, but this should be done only under the guidance of a physician.

Recommended dosage: 50 mg at bedtime. You can proceed to take 50 mg twice daily adding a capsule at breakfast. It can be taken with melatonin at bedtime if you have trouble falling asleep and staying asleep.

L-Tyrosine

L-Tyrosine plays an important role in the production of neurotransmitters that **regulate emotions** & also can help with **appetite suppression**.
L-tyrosine helps the brain to produce adequate amounts of the neurotransmitters L-dopa, dopamine, norepinephrine, & epinephrine.
If levels of these neurotransmitters are insufficient, feelings of **sadness, anxiety, irritability and frustration** can result.

In addition, dopamine helps suppress appetite and reduce body fat, so people with insufficient levels of this neurotransmitter may find **they are gaining weight or struggling to lose it.**

Other Benefits of L-Tyrosine
- Suppresses Appetite
- Increases Energy
- Enhances Libido
- Supports Thyroid Function
- Elevates Mood; Creates Feelings of Joy
- Increases Focus

Source: L-Tyrosine is found in protein containing foods, such as meats, dairy products, fish, wheat and oats.

Supplements: Take 500 mg 1 – 3 times per day

Fish Oils

Fish oils are essential for everyone to provide key omega-3 fatty acids (EPA & DHA)

Benefits:
- Studies have shown fish oils counteract depression
- Important for cognitive function & can prevent brain atrophy (shrinkage)

Other Important Benefits (improves symptoms of):
- Anxiety
- Bi polar disorder
- Brain health, Depression
- Fibrocystic breasts
- Dry Eyes
- Eczema / Itchy skin
- Fibromyalgia
- Arthritis Back Pain
- Mood
- Hair loss
- Heart Health
- High Blood Pressure
- High Cholesterol/Triglycerides
- Lupus
- Enlarged Prostate
- Seizure disorder
- Stroke Prevention
- Weight Loss
- Hormone balance
- ADD / ADHD

Everyone should be on a good fish oil supplement!

SO . . . my friends, you need to take your fish oils! Hate the taste? Take them before your meals to prevent any fish taste. Better yet, freeze them. This way the softgel will be in your intestines before it dissolves.

GABA & L-Theanine

What is GABA?
Gamma-aminobutyric acid is an amino acid found naturally in fish, especially mackerel, and wheat bran. Who eats enough of these? Not me! So supplementation is great.

What is L-Theanine?
It is an amino acid derivative found naturally in green tea. It creates a sense of relaxation and calming approximately 30-40 minutes after ingestion. Studies have demonstrated that L-Theanine helps increase alpha brain wave activity, **fostering a state of alert relaxation**. Studies have also shown L-Theanine **can be instrumental in weight loss** through regulating the brain's serotonin levels.

"GABA can restore brain function to youthful levels, help you lose weight, eliminate anxiety & reverse aging."
Eric Braverman M.D., neurologist, brain specialist

- Reduce Anxiety, Naturally
- Enhances Mood
- Relax without feeling drowsy
- Promotes better sleep
- Reverse brain deterioration / aging
- Increased mental alertness
- Eliminate cravings / food addictions
- Can help with ADD/ADHD
- Aids in weight loss

Suggested use: Take 550 mg of GABA & 200 mg of L-Theanine once or twice daily between meals or at the first signs of anxiety / stress.

I really like a product called Zen Mind which contains 550 mg of GABA and 200 mg of L-Theanine.

Progesterone

Progesterone crème is a natural anti-anxiety agent. I dislike flying and get very nervous beforehand. I will grab my jar of progesterone crème and slather it on. In about 7 – 15 minutes I'll get so relaxed, I will almost feel like I can fly the plane myself!

Fish Oils

See page 98.

See page 98.

Memory

Phosphatidylserine

Regain your Magnificent Memory! Promotes Brain Function, Brain Repair, Memory & Cognition.

What is Phosphatidylserine?

Phosphatidylserine is key in the maintenance of cellular function, particularly in the brain.

Benefits of PS:

- Best nutritional support on the market for memory
- Increases neuronal membrane fluidity (cell communication)
- Can prevent dementia & possibly Alzheimer's disease
- Improves memory loss due to aging
- Improves cognition
- Can alleviate stress-related anxiety
- Helps the brain retrieve information
- Helps with low energy in the morning
- Can correct either high or low cortisol levels

After only 2 weeks of use, users report a marked difference in their ability to:

- Remember
- Focus
- Speak with Clarity
- Feel Intelligence Return & Expand

I like one called PS100 by Jarrow Formulas which contains Phosphatidylserine (PS) 100 mg, phosphatidylcholine (PC) 12 mg, and Gamma tocopherol 3 mg.

This is one of my ALL-TIME favorites! I can't be without my PS. It's excellent for anyone over the age of 50.

Weight Loss

5-HTP
See page 96

L-Tyrosine
See page 97

SAM-e
See page 95

Libido

See Chapter 6

Insomnia

See Chapter 14

General Over-all Health

Vitamin D
For bones, breast health, depression, immune system

Why Am I Deficient?
- You don't spend enough time in the sun (almost all of us)
- You are over age 50

In fact, Vitamin D deficiency is almost epidemic!

Why should I take a Vitamin D supplement?
Vitamin D:
- Can reduce Breast Cancer risk
- Protects against cardio-vascular disease
- Can Protect against colds, flu & viral infections
- Boosts immune system
- Plays a strong role in bone health

- Low levels are linked with depression
- Low levels are associated with increased risk of Heart Attack 45%, Stroke 78%, and Premature Death 77%.
- Higher Vitamin D levels are associated with increased survival rates, including Breast Cancer survival.
- For Brain Power: Studies show good Vitamin D levels produce higher scores on memory tests

Wow! Now that's a comprehensive list of benefits.

How Much Vitamin D Do You Need?
Experts now agree that a dose of **2,000 – 4,000** IU is the daily amount needed to achieve optimal blood levels.

Milk Thistle
Tender, Loving Care for Your Liver!
The active ingredient in Milk Thistle is silymalin.
According to important studies, milk thistle extract can protect the cells of the liver by blocking the entrance of harmful toxins and helping remove these toxins from the liver cells.

Milk Thistle:
- Cleanses the liver
- Can stimulate production of new liver cells to replace older damaged cells
- Helps the body detox excess estrogens
- Can detox & protect the liver from toxic chemicals & pollutants

Almost everyone over the age of 50 should take milk thistle periodically because our livers are so over-taxed by pollutants, toxins and even the occasional alcoholic beverage. Baby your liver. You will feel more energetic!

Look for: Milk Thistle Seed 30:1 Extract 150 mg
Suggested use: Take 1 capsule per day

Worried About Family History of Cancer?
These Are Anti-cancerous

Vitamin D
- Toxic to cancer cells
- Increases P53 gene which targets & kills cancer cells
- Best dose: at least 1,000 IU per day

Milk Thistle
- Improves liver function
- Has anti-cancerous properties

Folate
- Decreases colon cancer up to 50%
- 400 mcg per day

Olive oil
- Contains anti-carcinogenic properties
- 2 tablespoons per day

Green tea
- Has potent anti-cancerous properties
- Increases calorie burning rate of the body. A nice added benefit!

There you go! I have been studying supplements for 30 years. These are the ones that are research-based & study-based. Just start with one or two. Don't go overboard or you won't know what is really working. Call me if you need help. I care about you!

"And the leaves of the tree were for the healing of the nations."
Revelation 22:2

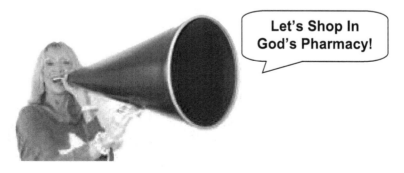

Let's Shop In God's Pharmacy!

Chapter 17

What About Exercise?
(The dreaded word for so many of you)

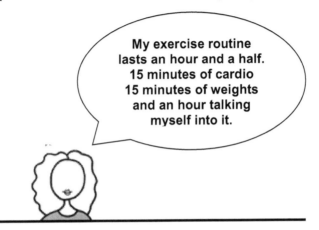

There are three reasons why people work out.
1) To improve their cardiovascular function and reduce risk of heart disease.
2) For fitness; in other words being able to lift the laundry basket or lift your suitcase or take the stairs instead of the elevator.
3) For weight loss.

I am definitely in favor of exercising to get yourself in better health. If you have heart disease or a family history of heart disease, then exercise is definitely going to be good for you.

Did you ever try to exercise when you are hungry or have not eaten enough calories?
You really can't do it, so you bulk up on calories so that you have enough energy to do the work out.
How will that work for weight-loss? It won't! Evidence about exercising not working for weight loss was reported in many studies that confirmed that exercise is useful in MAINTAINING weight loss, but it does NOT help people lose weight.

We have a proliferation of health clubs in the U.S. and people are just getting FATTER. We have basically seen a "fitness revolution" but we are still getting FATTER! Think about it.

But is exercise an important tool in weight-loss?
I have not seen evidence of that. My general attitude toward exercise is that is overrated as a tool for effective weight-loss.

In 2012, Herman Pontzer, a professor of anthropology reported his findings as to whether our sedentary lifestyle is to blame for the obesity epidemic.
Hunter found that our bodies adapt to account for our energy demands. He said if we push our bodies hard enough, we can increase our energy expenditure in the short term. But our bodies adapt and will eventually find ways to keep our over-all energy expenditures in check. In other words he concluded" we are getting fat because we eat too much not because we're sedentary" Pontzer concluded" we are not going to Jazzercise our way out of the obesity epidemic"

In fact, even faithful runners tend to get fatter as the years go by, even those that run more than 40 miles per week.
In truth, we do not burn a lot of calories by doing moderate exercise AND it often encourages us to eat more because we think we DID burn those calories.
If physical exercise was truly the answer, construction sites would be full of thin men. And you know that's not true!

Did you ever hear about people who exercise to "work up an appetite?" That's exactly what exercise can do. Your body wants to eat to replenish the energy you just spent. It's actually counter-intuitive.

Can Exercise Help Me Lose Weight?
As I said, studies show that exercise is good for staying fit, but is not the answer for losing weight. Most people who try to lose weight by exercise are also cutting out unhealthy foods. Did you ever see a regular jogger or aerobics buff eating a donut after they exercise?
No, they are more likely to be drinking some cool water or having something half-way healthy.

That's why these people can stay lean. If they eat the wrong foods, even the distance runner will gain weight.

Do You Hate To Exercise?
A recent large study about exercise divided dieters into 2 groups:
Group 1 Dieted only
Group 2 Dieted and exercised 45 minutes 3-5 days/week
The difference was ***only a couple of pounds***!
Diet only group lost 5 – 37 pounds.
Exercise/Diet group lost 8 – 39 pounds.

A compilation of over 43 studies have shown that exercise is not an effective weight loss tool. Of course it is important to your overall health, but walking is just fine.

> Forget "EAT LESS, EXERCISE MORE"
> **WHAT YOU SHOULD REALLY DO IS**
> **"EAT BETTER & WALK"**

Walking is great because it gets you into a healthful mood and it won't make you hungrier! A 20 minute daily walk is a great goal.

In a Nutshell:
Quite frankly, the main reason I believe in exercise is to maintain muscle and body tone and for heart health.
I do NOT believe in having to go to the gym to work off bad foods that I have eaten. I am not an extremely active person, but I have maintained my weight for many, many years without a scheduled exercise program.
My main form of exercise is walking, which I do every day. You do not need to be chained to a gym membership to maintain your desired weight.

Best Exercises For Those Of Us Over The Age Of 50

Arm Raises
Strengthen your shoulder muscles

1. Sit in a chair with your back straight.
2. Keep feet flat on the floor even with your shoulders.
3. Hold hand weights down at your sides with palms facing inward.
4. Raise both arms to side, shoulder height.
5. Hold the position for 1 second.
6. Slowly lower arms to the sides. Pause. Repeat 8 to 15 times.
7. Rest. Do another set of 8-15 repetitions.

Tricep Extensions
Strengthen muscles in the back of the arm.
So many women are concerned about the extra skin / fat on the back of their arms, so this exercise is your new best friend!

1. Sit near the front edge of a stable chair, feet flat on floor and even with shoulders.
2. Hold a weight in one hand, raise that arm straight toward the ceiling, palm facing in.
3. Support arm below the elbow with the other hand.
4. Slowly bend raised arm at elbow, bringing hand weight toward same shoulder.
5. Slowly re-straighten arm toward ceiling. Hold for 1 second.
6. Slowly bend arm toward shoulder again.
7. Pause, then repeat the bending and straightening until you have done the exercise 8-15 times. Repeat 8-15 times with other arm.
8. Rest. Then repeat a set of 8-15 repetitions on each side.

Brisk Walking For a Younger You
Walking is one fitness trend that never goes away!
A study of nurses found that walking 4 hours a week gave them a 41% lower risk of hip fractures, compared to walking less than an hour a week. 4 hours is not a lot. You can do it!

Maintain a pace that you can live with, but over and above that standard walk. The slower you go, the more you atrophy.

Do 'Unexpected' Exercises
Even the littlest bit of activity can go a long way toward keeping joints supple and muscles toned.

- Household-object resistance exercises. This is a great option for you. Common household items can be used for many excellent resistance exercises. For example, by simply squeezing a tennis ball or a small rubber ball, you can strengthen your grip and forearm muscles. A big book or a small paint can be used to do curls or overhead lifts. A chair can be used to strengthen your legs and lower back by doing multiple squats – sitting up and down – on it. Be creative and look around. You'll find lots of potential "exercise equipment" right around your house!
- Have a pool? Low-impact water workouts combine cardiovascular exercises with strength training, with little risk of injury. The added resistance of water makes the aerobics challenging. Water provides 12 times the resistance of air because of its density. As water pushes against the body, the movements become more difficult, requiring muscles to work harder. You can work out muscles in your upper and lower body just by making resistance movements underwater.
- Yard work exercises. This is the most overlooked fair-weather resistance exercise. Whether you mow the lawn, plant flowers, trim vines, fix a fence or do any of a thousand other outdoor duties, your yard is loaded with potential resistance exercises. But be careful of extreme weather conditions, which are common in the South and Midwest. Remember to regularly hydrate and use sunscreen, and don't overexpose yourself to the sun or heat.
- Outdoor activity exercises. There are many outdoor activities that can fall under the rubric of resistance exercise. From guided nature walks and kayaking to moderate hikes and biking. Again, if extreme weather conditions stay at bay.

God has given us an experiential playground on the planet that also serves as our global gym.

What About Weights?
You can purchase simple weights at almost any Walmart or similar store at low cost.

- Do strength exercises for all your major muscle groups **at least twice a week**, but vary the exercises so you don't work the same muscle group 2 days in a row.
- It's important to **gradually** add a challenging amount of weight in order to benefit from strength exercises. If you don't challenge your muscles, you won't get stronger. You can build up to using 1 or 2 pound weights as your strength grows and your body adapts to these strength exercises.
- Take 3 seconds to lift or push a weight into place. Hold the position for 1 second, and take another 3 seconds to lower the weight. Don't let the weight drop - lower it slowly.
- It should feel somewhat hard for you to lift or push the weight. If you can't lift or push a weight 8 times in a row, it's too heavy for you and you should reduce the amount of weight. If you can lift a weight more than 15 times in a row, it's too light for you. Increase the amount of weight.
- Do 8 to 15 repetitions in a row. Wait a minute, then do another set of 8 to 15 repetitions in a row of the same exercise.

I like weights and use them about 3 times per week . . . while I listen to the bible on tape.
A great resource is Daily Audio Bible. This is an app that you can have on your phone or computer. You can listen to the Word of our Lord on your headphones, in your car while driving, or listen to at home while doing your chores . . . It has broadcasts of the Bible designed to take you through the Bible in one year. This is one of my favorite benefits of new technology! You can find it at *dailyaudiobible.com*

Good Posture Is Very Important

My friend, a chiropractor says when you have proper posture, your spine is correctly aligned and this reduces your stress on your bones and your joints. So, aside from how it makes us look tall and strong, good posture has positive medical benefits.

So, shoulders back my friends.
Pretend you're in the army . . . stand up straight. Good posture immediately makes a man or woman appear younger AND more attractive.

And no shuffling gait. Pick up your feet, please. Next time you see a man or woman shuffling along, take note.
It totally ages you!

Don't be afraid of exercise, but don't be obsessed with it either. A Brisk Walk is Great!

> *"Do you not know that you are God's temple and that God's Spirit dwells in you? If anyone destroys God's temple, God will destroy him. For God's temple is holy, and you are that temple."*
>
> 1 Corinthians 3:16-17

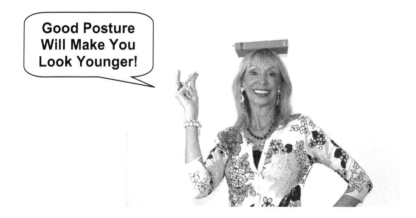

Good Posture Will Make You Look Younger!

Chapter 18

Barbara's Lifestyle Tips

Live Your Life Like A Younger You!
. . . No matter how old you are!

- Nourish the brain! Intellectual skills are NOT perishable
- Laugh a lot – laughing reduces stress. A good "belly laugh" actually raises those important serotonin levels. Get a book of one-liners, and help others laugh too.
- Create a regimen. Even if it's just the time you take to sit and read every day or sit outside in this sun. Regimens reduce anxiety, actually simplify your lifestyle and make life more enjoyable.
- Pickle Pick-Me-Up! Pickles flood brain cells with oxygen. Yes! Crunching on a pickle can chase away mental fatigue and brain fog within 60 seconds, according to scientists at UCLA. They found that the intense flavor combination of salt and tangy vinegar stimulates the central nervous system, which in turn increases blood flow to the brain. More energizing oxygen can reach your blood cells and perk you right up! We keep a large jar of pickles in the refrigerator at Better Health Naturally, for our afternoon pick-me-up! Try it and you will feel an instant 'zing' of energy.
- Smile, smile, smile. When my son was young, I taught him that when he smiles he should make it a MILLION DOLLAR smile. So beautiful! Takes years off your face.
- Stay excited life! If a new thing comes along, embrace the learning & knowledge. Don't turn into one of the people who scoffs "eh, technology" and talks about "The Old Days". Yikes . . . this turns you into one of "The Old Folks". Not for us! New things just fascinate us from now on. Listen to those "Young-uns" and try to be receptive instead of critical. There's still a lot we can learn.

Ladies:

- Opaque or texturized hose not only makes you look youthful but also hides leg veins
- Crème blush or gel blush on top of foundation gives a beautiful, healthy "Glow". Don't apply either of these over powder because you will get unsightly streaks. Powdered skin is aging . . . put away those powders.
- Get a pedicure every so often. Pretty toes make us feel youthful. Shy or embarrassed about your feet? Don't be! They've taken you far in life. Be proud of them, bunions & all!
- Jewelry: big jewelry is youthful. Think of the people you see on TV. They wear big earring, necklaces, rings and bracelets. PLUS costume jewelry is very inexpensive!
- Curl your eyelashes. So youthful! Dip your curler in warm water first. This creates a mini curling iron.
- At home Eye-Lift. Use an eye shadow at the outer corners of your eyes and swoop up toward outer brow. Instant lift!
- Nails: Having your nails done in a pretty color is very modern and makes you look well-groomed. It livens up our hands and makes them look fresh. You don't have to go to a salon. You can do it at home. Get yourself a nice creamy beige color or a nice beige-pink color. That way if you make a mistake and get outside the cuticle it's not hard to correct. Once in a while go bold. I like some deep purples and I also like red and coral for a change. We are never too old to have pretty colorful nails. My precious mother-in-law was 86 when she died and her little hands still had a pretty pink manicure.

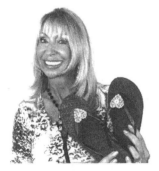

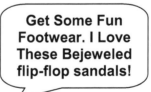

Get Some Fun Footwear. I Love These Bejeweled flip-flop sandals!

- Style: some things never go out of style, so wear them with flair. My mother-in-law LOVED palazzo pants and she rocked that style for years. I love things with fringe. They make me feel young & flirty. I also love wearing big rings. I don't worry about them going "out of style" because they are my style.

- Hats: Sometimes feel like you need to wear a hat? Maybe your hair is not up to snuff for the day? Or you just want to wear it for sun protection? Choose a hat that is flattering, NOT something your husband used to wear or something that looks like fisherman's hat. Get a stylish hat that suits the shape of your face. It does not have to be expensive. Maybe you look good in a Fedora or maybe you want to wear a wide brimmed hat. You only need one. The just-right hat can make you look very beautiful/handsome. I get so many compliments on the simple hat that my husband bought me. It just suits the shape of my face. It does not make me look dreary drab or old. In fact I feel quite buoyant when I wear it.

- Hydration: Don't like drinking water? I understand. Drink one glass every morning first thing when you wake up. The drink another full glass at lunch. Do the same thing just before dinner. There . . . now you have three nice glasses of water that will help you stay hydrated.

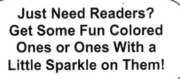

**Just Need Readers?
Get Some Fun Colored
Ones or Ones With a
Little Sparkle on Them!**

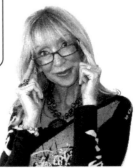

- Playfulness: Nothing makes you feel younger than acting playful. Is that difficult for you? Are you the serious type? Playfulness is not only state of body it is a state of mind. If you can't imagine what acting playful is like pretend you're playing with a puppy (Everyone knows how to do that) and transfer that into your state of mind and your joyfulness. Actors prove that is easy to simulate playfulness. They do it in their movies. When you act playful, even when you're not feeling playful, you will notice that you will eventually understand how that frame of mind makes you feel youthful. And then you will want to continue it. Hopefully!

"Pile your troubles on God's shoulders - he'll carry your load, he'll help you out. He'll never let good people topple into ruin."
Psalm 55:22

Chapter 19

The Younger You Happiness Factor
(A Surprising Study)

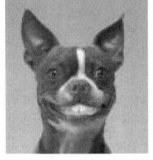

The Power of Positivity!

Okay, friends! It's time to perk up those smiles! Why? Studies are showing that people who smile more have better health. It's true! And it's not just a placebo. Sarah Pressman, an associate professor at UCI, recently proved that people who are happy and optimistic have a distinctive advantage over people who are angry, depressed, anxious or sad. How much of an advantage?

Her research has revealed that happy people contract less colds, post-surgery they have less pain and inflammation, they survive longer with lung cancer, they have less heart attacks (and when they do have heart attacks they die less frequently), they suffer fewer strokes, even their wounds heal faster! Happier people live longer!

How is it that happiness can have such an impact on our health?

It all comes down to stress. When your body is under stress your blood pressure, heart rate, stress hormones, cortisol levels and adrenaline all go through the roof!

This definitely takes a serious toll on your body. In other words, stress is killing you. No wonder depression is considered a contributing factor to heart attacks. Thankfully in Pressman's words, "Happiness is the anti-stress." Whenever you smile or have a moment of contentment, all those dangerous levels drop.

Now how difficult is it to find a simple of moment of contentment in your day? You can do it! People who have made happiness a state of being recover rapidly from stressful experiences. In the long term this leads to better immune function, a healthier body and an extended life!

Why it's Smart to Smile :)

So we know happiness leads to better health, but of course being happy is easier said than done. Thankfully your smile does NOT need to be genuine for you to feel the positive benefits. Don't believe us? Sarah Pressman recently did a smile study which is now famous. The Wall Street Journal, the New York Times and even Stephen Colbert are talking about Pressman's study and its incredible results!
Participants were divided into three groups and assigned stress-inducing tasks. One group performed the task without smiling, the second group had a fake smile, and the third had a genuine smile (what experts call a Duchenne smile). Surprisingly, both the fake smile AND the genuine smile groups had lowered heart rates and recovered quicker after completing their task. Outstanding!

This is great news for those you who struggle with depression or anxiety. Just start smiling! Even a "fake" smile will do. If your smile is not a result of genuine happiness, you will still experience lowered stress and better health! And who knows, if you make smiling a habit you may just start feeling more positive in general. Smile and the world smiles with you!

A Happy Lifestyle - More Benefits

Happiness has a greater impact on your health then purely as an anti-stress agent. People who have an optimistic attitude believe they have greater control over their own lives.

As a result they feel greater motivation to exercise, eat healthy and have regular doctor visits. Overall they take greater care of their body.

People who are happy are also less likely to take harmful drugs or smoke cigarettes, and without negative thoughts keeping them up at night, they sleep better! People who exude positive energy have more friends, richer social lives and more meaningful relationships with their family members.
Some of you may say, "Well, happiness is good and fine for those who don't have to worry about keeping a roof over their head and food on their table, but for the rest of us happiness is not our top priority!"

The Psychology Science Journal decided to put this belief to the test. Does happiness only benefit those who already have their basic needs met (i.e. they have shelter, food, medical care and safety)? Once again the results are surprising.
People in Third World countries who struggle daily with starvation, disease, poverty and violence show associations with happiness that are TWICE as strong compared to people who live comfortably.
This is shocking as it shows not only does happiness matter if you are struggling to have your basic needs met, it actually matters much more! Because the body is suffering as a result of lack of nutrition, no access to medicine, and the stresses of an unsafe lifestyle, the positive effects of happiness are more important and have a more dramatic effect on health.

So if you think you need to wait to get your life on track before making happiness a priority, think again! Happiness depends more on your state of mind then on external factors. Making an effort to achieve an optimistic perspective will have real and lasting mental and physical benefits on your health and well-being, even if you live in Somalia!
God is good and he wants you to live a life that's full of joy.

A YOUNGER YOU LIFE!

We at Better Health Naturally are here to help you! Feel free to call us anytime. We care not only about your physical health but your mental health as well. If you need help achieving a more positive mind set we want to help you get there! Remember we're your cheerleaders!
God is good and he wants you to live a life that's full of joy!

"Therefore with joy shall ye draw water out
of the wells of salvation."
Isaiah 12:3

Chapter 20

The Coffee Question
What about that "Cup o' Joe"?

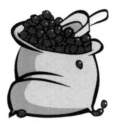

Hello Coffee Drinkers, Turns Out That You Are Really Smart!
To coffee or not to coffee? That is a favorite question.
Yes, I am a coffee drinker and I will tell you why!
Studies show up to 5 cups of coffee a day protects against many diseases.

Prostate Cancer
Men who drink at least six cups a day have a 60% lower risk of developing advanced prostate cancer than those who didn't drink any. The prostate cancer study compared the coffee-drinking habits of 50,000 men professionals with their incidence of prostate cancer over 20 years, and also took into account family history of prostate cancer and how frequently they had screenings. The more cups of coffee the men drank, the less likely they were to be in the most lethal group.

Diabetes
At least 18 studies have found that drinking three or more cups of coffee a day is linked with a lower risk of developing the disease. Studies show that people who drink three to four cups of java a day are 25% less likely to develop Type 2 diabetes than those who drink fewer than two cups. In both the prostate and diabetes studies, the health benefits were evident.

Coffee contains traces of hundreds of substances, including potassium, magnesium and vitamin E as well as chlorogenic acids that are thought to have antioxidant properties. These may protect against cell damage and inflammation that can be precursors to cancer, diabetes, neurological disorders and cardiovascular disease.

Parkinson's, Cirrhosis, Dementia, Cancer

Studies have shown that people who drink coffee regularly are 80% less likely to develop Parkinson's disease and liver cirrhosis. Two excellent studies done in 2009 have also suggested that drinking coffee lowers the risk of developing Dementia.

Many studies have also highlighted coffee's key role in reducing risk for multiple types of cancer. People who drink coffee are up to 50% less likely to develop liver cancer, while other research has also suggested that they are 25% less likely to develop colon cancer. Again, men who drink coffee have a 60% reduced risk of developing advanced prostate cancer.

Alzheimer's

Moderate daily consumption of caffeinated coffee may be an extremely valuable option for long-term protection against Alzheimer's memory loss. Coffee is inexpensive, easily gets into the brain, and appears to directly attack the disease process.

A new study shows that it may not be caffeine itself, but a combination of caffeine and coffee's compounds that together cause an increase in blood levels of a growth factor called GCSF (granulocyte colony stimulating factor). Patients with Alzheimer's disease have low levels of GCSF.

Top Five Reasons to NOT Quit Coffee

1. It protects your heart: Moderate coffee drinkers (1 to 3 cups/day) have lower rates of stroke than non-coffee drinkers, an effect linked to coffee's antioxidants. Coffee has more antioxidants per serving than blueberries, making it the biggest source of antioxidants in American diets.

Immediately after drinking it, coffee raises your blood pressure and heart rate, but over the long term, it can actually lower blood pressure as coffee's antioxidants activate nitric oxide, widening blood vessels.

2. It prevents diabetes: These antioxidants boost your cells' sensitivity to insulin, which helps regulate blood sugar.
3. Your liver loves it: It appears that the more coffee people drink, the lower their incidence of cirrhosis and other liver diseases. An analysis of nine studies found that every 2-cup increase in daily coffee intake reduced liver cancer risk by 43%.
4. It boosts your brain power: Drinking between 1& 5 cups a day may help reduce risk of dementia and Alzheimer's disease, as well as Parkinson's disease. Those antioxidants may ward off brain cell damage and help the neurotransmitters involved in cognitive function to work better.
5. It helps headaches: Studies show that 200 milligrams of caffeine – about the amount in 16 ounces of brewed coffee – provides relief from headaches, including migraines.

Now, you can sit back with a freshly brewed cup and be comforted by the fact that you no longer have to feel guilty about it.

YAY! I LOVE coffee!

"And God said, Behold, I have given you every plant yielding seed that is on the face of all the earth, and every tree with seed in its fruit. You shall have them for food."
Genesis 1:29

Part II

Looking Like The

Younger You

Chapter 21

Let Your Skin Bloom Like A Rose

As we age, collagen breaks down. Skin begins to sag, wrinkle and lose elasticity. It can become rough, dry or blotchy. Your hormones have changed and so has your skin.
The GLOW is gone . . . but NOT for good!
Don't be afraid to layer your products. It's impossible to get all the wonderful anti-aging agents in one product.

Let's look at your skin type and find what will be best for YOUR "Younger You".

(New Healthy Skin product recommendations can be found in parentheses).

White / Light Skin
White skin is typically thinner than other skin types and has less melanin.
- Be careful of the sun. Use a moisturizer with SPF 15 (Daytime Moisturizer with SPF15)
- White skin is prone to Rosacea. If this is an issue with you, Ester C can be most helpful ("C" U-Later Wrinkles)
- Microdermabrasion or acid peels are okay as white skin does not scar easily.

Brown / Dark Skin
Brown skin has high melanin which can trigger the release of chemicals that attach & break down elastin. Your skin needs TLC!
- Brown skin tends to be more oily
- It is more susceptible to inflammation & acne
- Avoid lasers, deep peels, & microderm treatments because you are more susceptible to scaring.
- AHA (glycolic acid) treatment is fine but avoid prescription Retin-A that can discolor skin.

Asian / Yellow Skin

Asian skin has excessive amounts of melanin which gives your skin its beautiful yellow undertones. Which, incidentally, protects you against skin cancer.

- Your skin will show discolorations, dark spots, freckles, and hyperpigmentation before wrinkles & loss of skin elasticity.
- You are more prone to acne as your skin produces more oil, which can clog pores & cause breakouts
- You are sensitive & prone to irritation, so avoid skin care products with fragrance.
- Pores can be larger than other ethnicities, therefore exfoliation should be part of your daily routine. Larger pores have a higher susceptibility of getting clogged.
- Cleanse your skin 2 times per day with oil-free, fragrance-free cleanser. Exfoliate 2 times per week for beautiful, healthy skin.
- Rejuvenate T.R. and Retin-AL are also recommended.

Specific Skin Conditions

Fine lines and wrinkles

Fine Lines & Wrinkles are a result of age-related weakening of the skin's collagen and elastin, the fibers that keep skin FIRM.

To Rebuild Collagen and Elastin

1. Choose an Ester C product ("C" U-Later Wrinkles). Ester-C is proven to stimulate collagen production and can dramatically reduce wrinkles.
2. Use a Retinol product (Retin-AL) which works on both fine lines & deep wrinkles. "C" U-Later works from the inside out; Retinol works from the outside in.
3. A peptide product is also great for you.

Skin Discoloration & The Dreaded Age Spots

Blotches, in which small patches of skin appear to have a different color than the main skin area, become common as we age. The skin will not reflect light and you can look older than a person who has even more lines & wrinkles than you. UV exposure can cause the melanin in our skin to cluster into brown spots in African American, Asian or Hispanic skin.

To Correct Spots & Blotching
1. Use a good bio-identical progesterone crème such as ProHELP / Menopause Moisture Crème
2. Use an Ester-C product to even out your skin tone.
3. Use a glycolic acid product AFTER the "C" product.
4. You can add a Retinol product, the purest form of Vitamin A (Retin-AL). This evens skin tone & gives a rosy glow.
5. If necessary, add a skin bleaching product directly on prominent or stubborn spots. Kojic acid works best.
6. For deep (dermal) pigmentation, photo-laser treatment can be an adjunctive therapy.

For a nice even skin tone, wear a sunscreen containing SPF 15 daily. In very hot climates, SPF 30 is even better.

Thinning Skin
The skin of older individuals often becomes papery thin. As the stratum corneum thickens, the epidermis & dermis gets thinner. Oil gland activity declines. This can also be due to hormonal decline.

To Improve Elasticity
1. Use a bio-identical progesterone crème such as ProHELP or Menopause Moisture Crème.
2. Use a Retinol product to increase cellular strength and new cell development deep within the skin. (Retin-AL)
3. A DMAE product is great as it "Lifts" the skin (Lift-In-A-Jar).

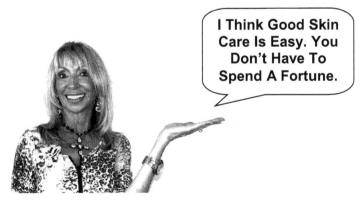

I Think Good Skin Care Is Easy. You Don't Have To Spend A Fortune.

Dry / Dull Skin

As we age, skin becomes drier. Up to age of 14, the skin on the face exfoliates naturally every 14 days. This quick rate of renewal leaves youngsters with a healthy-looking, glowing complexion. By age 45 the skin will only exfoliate every 28 days or so. The resulting build-up of dead skin cells can leave the skin looking dull or grey.

To Hydrate Dry Skin

1. Exfoliate the outer layer of the skin either by buffing and/or with a glycolic acid product. Cleansers with micro-beads will gently exfoliate the skin and remove dead skin cells and uncover glowing skin beneath. **It is a myth that exfoliation makes skin dryer.** People with dry skin have more loose dead cell layers than others and therefore MUST exfoliate. (Buffing Pearls Cleanser is great).
2. Use an AHA glycolic acid product. AHA stands for Alpha Hydroxy Acid. The best form is glycolic acid which is made from sugar cane. (Rejuvenate T.R.) It penetrates the deep dermal layers to bring about the most dramatic changes.

What Can Glycolic Acid Do For You?

- Removes build-up on top layers of the skin
- Allows healthier cells to come to the surface
- Vastly improves skin's texture and color
- Has water binding properties, retains moisture in skin, increasing hydration
- Improves effectiveness of all other skin care

For Extra Moisture: Hyaluronic Acid (Advanced Hydration Complex) is an amazing moisturizer; the best I have ever found and I have looked high & wide.

Rough Skin

Rough skin is commonly caused by the accumulation of dead skin cells on the skin's surface. This causes the skin surface to appear bumpy and rough. Complexion will appear dull & lifeless.

To Smooth Skin
1. Use a Retinol product—lessens roughness as well as blotches. (Retin-AL)
2. Use Glycolic Acid (Rejuvenate T.R.).
3. Hyaluronic Acid (Advanced Hydration Complex). This fabulous ingredient will make skin soft & smooth.

Acne
Acne is caused by a disorder of the sebaceous glands which block pores. This produces pimples or blemishes.

To Treat & Prevent Acne
1. Glycolic acid unclogs pores and minimizes their appearance (Rejuvenate T.R). Glycolic acid can also reduce acne scarring and prevent future acne.
2. Benzoyl Peroxide has AMAZING anti-acne properties. BP is the "gold standard" for treating acne. Vivant Skin Care has a great BP acne line that we carry.
3. Consider using a toner after cleansing, and before applying other products. It clears skin of any residual contaminants.

Thin Lips
DMAE applied directly on the lips can make them fuller & also give a lift to above-the-lip skin in a very short time. (DMAE is found in our Lift-In-A-Jar). You can feel it working.

Dark line along upper lip?
Use ester C serum & a bleaching cream. You'll be amazed!

Enlarged Pores
- Glycolic acid (Rejuvenate TR) reduces size of large pores
- Buffing Pearls Cleanser is excellent for diminishing pores.

Sagging Skin / Jaw Line
Take a 2-pronged approach.
- Choose a Vitamin C product like *"C" U-Later Wrinkles.* Facial contours will begin to appear tighter.

- Products containing DMAE (Lift-In-A-Jar) can actually re-define facial contours. Smooth on face and neck with upward strokes. Can also be used on tip of nose, upper eyelids and above lips!

Eyes: Dark Circles / Fine Lines
- Research has shown Haloxyl (a natural enzyme complex) reduces under-eye circles and reduces fine lines (Firm & Fade Eye Cream).
- Vitamin C, particularly Ester C, can stimulate collagen in the under-eye area.
- Vitamin C also brightens the area under the eye.

Rosacea
- Glycolic Acid is very helpful (Rosacea is a disease of reaction, not sensitivity, so using acids is fine)
- A good Vitamin C product - reduces redness and reduces dilated capillaries ("C"-U-Later Wrinkles) Valerie's Secret Rosacea contains Hyaluronic Acid, Aloe Vera, Vitamin E, and Green Tea which all help rosacea
- Avoid products containing botanical ingredients which can cause reactions

Scar Reduction
- A scar is a loss of tissue.
- Glycolic improves mild to moderate scarring; it lightens the interior surface of the scar. Results can be dramatic!
- Ester "C" can help stimulate collagen
- Try a product containing Aloe Vera which has given people great results

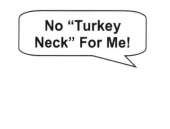

No "Turkey Neck" For Me!

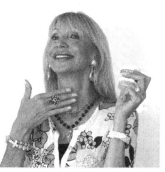

Dark spots where you had scarring?
Purchase some Vitamin K capsules, puncture and apply to bruised area. This will diminish scarring. Or look for a Vitamin K crème.

Neck
What ever you do to your face, do the same to your neck!
- DMAE smoothes & firms
- Use a bleaching serum, cream or lotion for any age spots to reverse them and/or prevent them from getting darker

Men's Skin Care

Men, Step Up to the Skin Care plate!
Men, I invite you to take special care of your face. Why? It's the first thing people notice. Wouldn't you want to make a great first impression? Well I'm going to give you some helpful tips so you can have wonderful skin.

Summer heat can be especially harsh on your facial skin, so you need to take precautions. Having a great facial cleanser is important. This rinses away dirt, oil, and impurities. It cleans deep in your pores and exfoliates, leaving a brighter complexion, and a fresh rejuvenated look.

After cleansing and shaving, rinse off with warm "never hot" water, to avoid dryness. Apply a toner with ingredients that are going to hydrate. We like toners with glycolic and lactic acids. Enriched with witch hazel, dissolves dead skin cells and clears contaminants.
If you are more on the oily side, I recommend skipping the toner.

Men, let's get you started on an age defining regimen that you can use daily. An Ester-C serum is excellent for men. The appearance of fine lines, wrinkles, and age spots are lessened. It can increase elasticity and even out skin tone. Most importantly, ester-C hydrates and firms wrinkle lines.

I believe that it is extremely important is to have a moisturizer that will hydrate your skin as well as protect it. An SPF of at least 15 will protect skin against premature aging, including age/sun spots, blotches and wrinkles.

Follow these simple tips to have the best skin you've had in years. Have luminous skin that makes you feel and look 10 years younger. You may be shocked at your results. If you think you're too much of a macho-man to care about your skin, you're not. Make yourself into a "handsome macho-man!" This can enhance your confidence in your overall appearance, making you feel like you can take on the world "Face First".

Summary of The Best Active Ingredients

Glycolic Acid – Removes dead cells from the surface of skin. Can reverse sun damage. Glycolic acid is key to luminous skin. Look for a 10% glycolic product.

Exfoliants – Remove dead cells & debris

Ester C – Rebuilds collagen. Can help smooth out fine lines and wrinkles. Evens out pigmentation. Can reduce or eliminate brown spots or freckles.

Vitamin A – Promotes cell turnover and new cell production and promotes more even texture

DMAE – Has a dramatic firming effect and is used by plastic surgeons as a disfiguration treatment. Studies showed significant improvement in overall appearance of aging skin, forehead lines, coarse wrinkles, eye area, lip area & smile lines, and sagging skin. When DMAE is applied topically it begins to work within minutes of application and continues to firm the skin over time.

Vitamin E – Repairs cells & tissue, promotes moisture

Peptides – The building blocks of proteins, penetrate the epidermis and send signals to cells, rebuilding diminished elasticity and firmness for more youthful looking skin. They work in a different manner than Ester-C which rebuilds collagen.

Hyaluronic Acid – A natural element in healthy skin, acts as a superior water-binding ingredient. It locks moisture into fluid-heavy spaces between cells.

Retinol – Stimulates collagen and elastin production to help prevent the signs of aging. Elasticity is restored; skin looks smoother & younger. Our Retin-AL product also contains Matrixyl, a peptide complex that is proven to reduce wrinkle density, depth, & volume.

<u>Barbara's Best Skin Care Tips</u>

At Nighttime
At night, choose a product either with retinol or collagen building peptides. Nighttime is a great time to apply serums since you won't be putting makeup on over them.

Exfoliation
As we age, dead skin cells stich together and stay on the skin much longer than when we were in our 20's.
Exfoliation removes those dead cells and increases production of new healthy cells. This is why I created the New Healthy Skin Buffing Pearls Cleanser with gentle exfoliating beads.
Exfoliate at least twice per week to look younger and dewier.
Is your skin already smooth and glowing? You can kick it up a notch. How? Give yourself an at home peel.
You can either use a Microdermabrasion cream (I like Clinician's Complex) or super-strength glycolic product (up to 20%). Leave the glycolic acid on for 2 to 5 minutes. This will really give you a wonderful result. Use once or twice a week.

Serums
Serums go on before creams. Your serum will not be able to penetrate as well through the thicker cream.

I love Retinol serum products (Vitamin A derivative). They speed up cell renewal, make skin tone more even and can reverse sun damage. Great for acne too.

Facial masks
Masks have been around since Cleopatra's days and now they have the benefit of being inexpensive and safe and anything but old-fashioned.

I love facial mask for mature skin. They help to tighten the skin nourish your collagen and firm your skin. They can also exfoliate if you choose an exfoliating mask. They will also help in enlarged pores and dry skin Dan there are wonderful before you're going out 20 event to make your skin look dewy and moist.

I recommend you use a mask on your skin at least once a week man joke for you it's calming and soothing and you'll notice an immediate result in the texture and brightness of your skin

Here is one of my favorites:
Hyaluronic Hydrating Mask by Derma e this wonderful mask will plump and hydrate your skin, diminishes the appearance of fine lines and wrinkles. It deeply hydrates dry, thirsty skin leaving it smoother softer and younger looking and it's an award winning formula. This is what I like to call a date mask. Apply it before you go out to an event.
Whenever I use my hydrating mask people usually comment that my skin looks wonderful.

It gives deep, deep hydration. Yum! A pricey alternative is dermatologic multivitamin power recovery mask. Phenomenal, but pricey. Cost is over $45 for a 2.5 ounce tube. But if you get it you could alternate it and use it maybe every other week and use the Hyaluronic Hydrating Mask on the other alternate week.

Eat Right!
Refined carbs cause insulin spiking which causes body to accumulate advanced glycation end products known as AGEs. These disrupt your skin's collage & elastin.
So . . . lose those "FRANKENcarbs". For more help, read my book, Eat Yourself Slender. You can also write or call my office for some free written information.

Conclusion
It's really not complicated.
Find your pressing skin issue & address it with good, affordable products. Sometimes one or two products can dramatically change the look or your skin. If you like to use a lot of products, don't be afraid to layer. We can't put every key or active ingredient in the same base . . . they often require different delivery systems or base ingredients.
I call it "layering technology", and I layer a lot!
You can look as young as you feel. I promise!

"She is more precious than jewels, and nothing you desire can compare with her."
Proverbs 3:15

Chapter 22

Make-up For The Younger You: Apply Yourself, Ladies

One of the worst mistakes we women can make as we grow older is to wear outdated or old-fashioned make-up.
We want to look fresh. Here is how!

I am not saying that just by putting a different makeup on or lipstick it's going to have a profound effect on your life. But taking a little extra time to make sure you feel good before you walk out the door will make you feel more confident, prettier and add a bit of spring to your step and that's what I want for you! The youthful attitude will accompany the look.
Taking the time to find the right products really pays off. Are you in a rut with your make-up regimen? Time to break out! AND my goal for you is 15 minutes and out the door!
ALSO: good make-up, like good skin care doesn't have to cost a lot! Don't go for the splurge . . . Go for "the steal" (bargain).

All ingredients are not created equal. When we purchase ingredients for our skin care products, there are different grades, and that completely affects the products. Also, the ingredients should be formulated in a way that is effective so they will transform your skin.

Foundation
Glowing Makeup Made Easy
Self-tanners are great for a sun-kissed glow. I'm a big fan! I like Clarins Liquid Bronze Self Tanner. After you apply it, use a Q-tip to swipe any dark spots on your face so they don't get darker. I also like Jergens Natural Glow Daily Facial Moisturizer, it gradually creates a natural looking glow and contains UVA / UVB SPF 20.

If you wear heavier makeup on a daily basis, when you are just around the house use only a tinted moisturizer & lip gloss or a nice hydrating lipstick.

Choose a fresh, light reflecting formula for a dewier look. Heavy foundations highlight lines & wrinkles and makes us look older. If a sales girl tells you that you need a heavier foundation just say NO!
A tinted moisturizer is my favorite for ladies over the age of 40. If you do nothing else to update your makeup or start wearing makeup for the first time, let it be a tinted moisturizer with SPF. You get 3 in 1 benefits – Moisturizer, Foundation & Sunscreen. So pretty! Tinted moisturizers are very youthful. For a bit heavier coverage mix with another form of foundation that you already have.
Choose a nice warm shade.

Concealer

Choose a "dual" concealer with 2 shades. First apply the lighter shade, then top with the darker shade.
Noticeable dark circles? You need a yellow based concealer, yellow cancels out purple tones. No matter what color skin you have – from very pale to dark brown – concealer should be one or two shades lighter than your skin.
I always dab concealer on the interior corner of the eye. People just put it in that half-moon of skin under the eye, but that interior spot can get quite shadowy and tired. If you have darker skin, put just a touch of gold eye shadow there; if you have lighter skin, use a touch of something shell-like.

Bronzer

I Love bronzer. I use it all year to warm up my complexion. Apply to cheek bones and around the outlines of your face, across chin & across forehead. I LOVE our collage powder, Soliel. It offers the best variety of shades of bronze with holographic pigments that blend together for bronzing, highlighting, and evening out skin tones. Creates a soft and youthful glow; the perfect California, sun-kissed look.

Eye Shadow

Don't think you can't have fun doing your eyes as you get older.
Cream eye shadows create bright and dewy eyes. Look for a neutral shade with just a hint of shimmer. All that's required to give the impression of a full eight hours of sleep to tired eyes is a quick swipe of cream onto the lids, smoothed with the fingers into a thin layer. You can also blend it right up to the brow bone. So gorgeous!
Eyes that sparkle instantly rejuvenate you. Dab a warm, light color shadow like gold or shimmery beige underneath the arch of your brow. Instant eye lift!
I also love a smoky eye. It can define eyes, make them "pop" and draw attention away from lines.

Eye Liner

Nothing is more important in making eyes POP than eyeliner. Eyes appear larger and more vibrant. A pencil is the easiest kind of eyeliner to apply. Start with a thin line at the inner corner of the eye and gradually thicken the line as you move to the outer corner. If you also use eyeliner under your eyes, make it a thinner line.
Use soft pencils that don't pull skin. Personally, I always line my eyes, even on weekends, even if I'm not wearing any other makeup. I'm addicted to the youthful look of "bigger" eyes.

Lashes

If your lashes are thin, mascara is your best beauty secret! There is no need for thin lashes in this age of cosmetics.
1-2 coats of mascara will make your eyes look larger, brighter and yes, even sexier! I have been using various mascaras since I was 18 years old and don't believe mascara needs to be expensive. You can have gorgeous lashes at an affordable price.

Look for a mascara that has keratin or a conditioner in it. This nourishes the lashes. No more brittle, dry lashes that fall out!
I use a combination conditioning, lengthening mascara. Longer lashes make you look more youthful then thicker lashes do.

Should you curl your lashes?
Curl them if you have time. Eyes look brighter and younger because more of your whites are exposed. Hold curler for 15 seconds. Voila! Movie star eyes for you.

Lips
No matte lipsticks! Choose a hydrating formula. I like to use a DMAE product on my lips once a day for plumpness and lift. Matte lipstick can end up looking dry and crumbly. Look for a satiny finish or use a gloss over your matte shades. Don't throw everything out . . . use what you've got, just "youthinize" it by mixing it with a little moisturizer or gloss before applying.

What color lipstick?
Light, rosy skin: soft pink
Light skin, yellow undertones: coral, peach
Medium rosy: violet grape, plum
Medium, yellow undertones: bluish reds
Dark skin: Red, coral, even a pretty brownish tint

To enhance lips & prolong color:
- Draw a line just outside of lips with a neutral color or lighter color that the lipstick you will be wearing
- Fill lips in with the same pencil
- Apply moisturizing lipstick over the pencil

Live in a hot climate?
Keep you lip liners in the refrigerator for a more precise line.

I love a product that is a stain and gloss all-in-one. I have one called Cranberry in the Younger You line and I get many compliments when I wear it!

There are some wonderful "lip plumpers" on the market that you can purchase that really work. I've listed one in the appendix. Personally, I dab DMAE cream on my lips every morning. It really does the job of a plumper and doubles as my "lift" product on other areas of my face.

Cheeks

I don't leave the house without my blush on. I use a peachy or pink color and sometimes one with a little bit of shimmer. Crème blushes leave a dewy, youthful finish. Great for dry skin too. Look glamorous & natural at the same time. Rosy, creamy colors will make you look blooming and chic and up-to-date.

Brow

To define brows use a neutral colored eyebrow pencil like taupe. Or use a powder and brow brush. Don't go too dark as that's only for the young'uns, otherwise it makes us look older.

What Kind of Brow?

Long face – Slight arch. Place arch outside edge of iris. Point end toward top of ear.

Square face – Centered arch. Above pupil. Point end toward center of ear.

Round face – Very high arch. Above pupil. Make end short, directly above ear.

Oval face – Brow straight, without much arch. Slight arch just outside the iris. End pointing toward middle of the ear.

My Best Beauty Regimen

Step 1: Conceal & Lighten
Dab Duo Corrector on under-eye area or any dark skin discoloration or your own concealer.

Step 2: Youthful Eyes
A) Apply a thin layer of crème eye shadow for some glow.
B) Add some "POP" with eyeliner.
C) Finish with a coat of lengthening or keratin mascara.

Step 3: Creamy Glowing Skin
Apply Tinted Moisturizer with SPF to entire face.

Step 4: Youthful Blush
Rub a dab of creamy blush on the apples of your cheeks for a beautiful glow.

Step 5: Lips
Use a luscious lip stain (color + gloss all-in-one) or use a lip enhancer for plump, luscious, hydrated lips.

<u>Reminder:</u> Don't stress over your make-up. It always looks younger and more flattering to be a little bit underdone.

If you have great skin, a dewy foundation, a nice blush and a "rockin" color lipstick you can pretty much do whatever else you want. Those are the things that make people say, "Oh, you look great!"

If you have a drawer full of make-up you rarely use, try blending a few products (your own little chemistry lab). If you need help, call me. I LOVE playing with make-up!

"The King is enthralled by your beauty."
Psalm 45:11

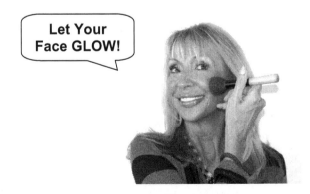

Let Your Face GLOW!

Chapter 23

Hair Care For The Younger You

Are you having an Old Hair Day or YEAR?
Here are my best tips!

Nourish, Nourish, Nourish!
Dry hair looks old. Conditioner makes all the difference. Purchase the best conditioner you can find in your price range. I really love one that is called Moroccan Oil. The actual Moroccan Oil brand is very exclusive and quite expensive. However, you can now find products containing Moroccan oil in local drugstores. Your hair will glow and be shiny and you will feel 10 years younger. Nourishment works for the entire body, including hair.

Hair Style – Make It Youthful
Men usually don't have this problem but we girls can develop what I call "old lady hair" as we age. I'm referring to our haircuts. You don't need to be trendy or faddish. Just get a great haircut that suits the shape of your face once every few months or so if you can afford it. If not, as you can fit it into your budget. This will make such a difference in creating a chic and youthful look.

If you want short hair, go short but keep it a slight bit shaggy. This will help you look modern and up to date. Also, the shaggy look makes it appear that you have more hair.

You don't need to get a haircut every six weeks. As a matter of fact longer hair is more youthful looking. That's why many older celebrities have longer hair. I keep mine quite long and I am well over the age of 50. If you keep your hair shiny and well-cut you will definitely feel younger. Don't lapse into "old lady" hair.

By the way, if you were born in my generation your mother may have told you to brush your hair 100 strokes a night. This is not a good idea as it will pull hair out of its follicles and can weaken individual strands. For brushing, use a nice boar bristle brush. It's gentlest on your hair.

Thin Hair
For thicker-looking hair, I like products called root-boost or root lifters. These have an ingredient that coats the hair and makes the root stand up on end. Another trick is to flip your head upside down when you are blow drying it. That will keep the root in the lifted position.

Do You Get The "Frizzies"?
Use a silkening serum. Smooth, sleek hair will shave years off your life. NO over-perming for you. Get just a light body wave every   12-16 weeks or so.

How often should you shampoo your hair?
If you have oily hair, shampoo every day. If your hair is normal wash every other day. If your scalp is dry, wash every few days. Don't feel guilty . . . resting your hair allows natural oils to build up & restore health.

For dry hair, look for a moisturizing shampoo. Find one that doesn't contain sodium laurel sulfate which can dry both your scalp and hair.

After menopause hair loses some of its oil in that case you may need to switch to a shampoo that is different from the one you were used to using.
Pantene makes some VERY nice products that are quite reasonably priced.

There are some excellent dry shampoos on the market that you could use alternatively with your regular shampoo. Dry shampoos have come a long way! These are designed to soak up any dirt in your hair. You then brush them out. Usually, this will also give you very nice volume.

My favorites are a dry powder shampoo by Oscar Blandi, called Pronto Dry Shampoo. Also, a Dry shampoo spray by Rene Furterer, called Naturia Dry Shampoo with Absorbant Clay.

By The Way . . .
If you were born in my generation you were taught that you should shampoo your hair twice to get it really clean. This is a myth. One application of shampoo is more than enough to adequately cleanse the scalp and hair.

Should I use a conditioner if I have thin or limp hair?
Yes, definitely. In fact, you need it more than most people because if hair is not conditioned, it is more likely to break.

Don't forget to put your conditioner all the way down to the roots of your hair. I like to alternate a conditioner with a deep conditioning treatment, sometimes called a hair masque.

Hair care tips for the "Younger You"
- Don't frost - the look is not natural. Go for subtle highlights instead. The crown and directly around the face are most youthful places to add highlights.
- Don't get a tight perm. Loose curls are youthful.
- Hide forehead lines with bangs. Not thick ones, they should be "wispy" & texturized. Not too short.
- Use the best conditioner you can afford. Your hair will look 100% better – shiny, rich & hydrated.
- Want Some Extra Shine?
  Consider a shine – enhancement product. There are wonderful shine serums or shine sprays that you can use. They reflect light off your hair. You don't need much. This investment can last a LONG time.

May your hair look as young as you on
the Younger You program.

No "old lady" hair for you!

Hair Care Tips Especially for the Men

Don't Be Rough!

Treat wet hair with special care. Hair's main component is a protein called keratin. Water stretches and weakens keratin molecules, so hair is more fragile when wet.

To minimize damage, wash hair only as needed. If you have naturally oily hair, that may be daily, but most guys can go longer.

Over-washing can actually dull hair by stripping away protective oils.

Make your routine as gentle as possible. Massage the scalp rather than scrubbing, and blot hair dry with a towel instead of firing up the blow dryer. To properly towel dry, shake out the excess water and stroke your hair in the direction it grows, rather than rubbing. Drying takes a bit longer this way, but you will soon notice the difference in the way your hair looks . . . less frizzy and less split ends. If you blow dry, apply a thermal styling spray or conditioner.

One more thing, don't shampoo with water that is too hot. It causes dry scalp as it strips essential oils from the skin.

Watch the Greasy Stuff

Gels and other styling aids create some nice looks, but be careful. Gels contain polymers -- that is, plastic -- dissolved in alcohol. Alcohol can weaken keratin and strip hair of moisture & oil, leaving hair weak and brittle. Use gels sparingly, preferably those that are alcohol free.

Also, go easy on the pomades and waxes which contain heavier ingredients like petroleum jelly and beeswax. Removing them may take repeated washings or a stronger shampoo than you would otherwise use, which can also damage hair.

Get a Good Haircut

Once hairs sprout from your scalp, it's no longer growing – just growing older. Hair on the end of a strands has seen a lot of wear and tear. Also, hair naturally loses moisture with age.

The cuticle can split at the end causing further weakness, dryness & damage.

A regular trim helps nip the problem in the bud. Hair strength varies with genes, washing routine and other treatments, and exposure to sun and heat, so some guys can go longer between cuts than others. Because the cuticle reflects light, dull hair is a sign that the cuticle is cracking. Act soon to avoid a head full of frizzies.

Oily Hair

The oil found in your hair is called sebum, and it is produced by the sebaceous glands in your scalp for the sole purpose of moisturizing your scalp. Hair that becomes too oily is the result of the over activity of the sebaceous glands, which can be caused by stress, a hormonal change, or poor diet with lots of oily foods.

- Wash your hair less. Yes, that's right! Shampoos are designed to strip the oils from your hair and scalp. Shampooing too often makes your scalp dry, and your scalp will work overtime to replace the oils lost. You've just made the problem worse!
- Be gentle: Vigorous brushing and scrubbing while shampooing also stimulate the sebaceous glands to produce more oils.
- Switch shampoos: There is nothing wrong with Head and Shoulders, but in your case, you suffer from oily hair, not dandruff. Use a clarifying shampoo that has a mild pH instead.
- If you are blow-drying your hair, limit the length of time the heat is on your scalp. Long exposure to heat on the scalp also stimulates the sebaceous glands to produce oil.

Balding / Thinning hair

DHT is a byproduct of the hormone testosterone and is the culprit in male pattern baldness. There are several changes in lifestyle that contribute to the reduction of DHT in your body and therefore indirectly can lead to the stimulation of hair growth. Progesterone can limit production of DHT.

Studies also show that the consumption of caffeine and herbal supplements such as green tea and ginkgo biloba have a direct effect on stimulating hair growth as well.

As hair starts to grow, consider purchasing a thickening shampoo, and then later on, a styling product (hair putty is a good one) for greater fullness and texture. There are also products called "hair putty" that give greater fullness and texture for you.

A good way to hide thinning hair is to try a new hairstyle. Consider a scissor-cut hairstyle, short to medium length. If you can see scalp on top, cut the sides short enough to expose an equal amount of scalp. This balances you and minimizes the appearance of balding. This will allow you to style your hair with a hair paste or putty and make your hair look fuller. When the sides and back are worn longer, it makes the top appear thinner. If you've lost a great deal of hair and this suggestion won't work, your next realistic choice would be to get a low buzz cut; this way your hair can blend easier with those thinning areas. It's perfect for keeping everyone's eyes on your face instead of your bald spot.
Look for a volumizing shampoo and conditioner that can add thickness and fluffs.
Also, see Chapter 8 for hair thinning or hair loss.

Get the Right Haircut / Style
Need a change? A big hair mistake is wearing hairstyles that do not fit your face. This is also why a goatee can look great on one man, but not another. Your haircut and facial hair need to be complementary to your face shape. A good barber will guide you in the right direction.
Search the Internet and magazines for a look that you feel best suits you. Pick your top two or three. Then take the pictures to your barber. You may walk out a new man!

Massage Your Scalp
Scalp massages helps promote good blood flow to the scalp, soothe nerves and relax muscles. Scalp massage also helps hair growth and luster. It feels great, too. Once each week,

massage the scalp with the fingertips using a firm pressure in a circular motion. Place the fingers under the hair to avoid pulling. Massage for about three minutes.

Gray Hair: Should I Color?
Coloring gray will be a routine that will need to be maintained at least once a month and often, twice. Because men wear their hair shorter than most women, the gray hairs become noticeable more quickly. This could challenge your budget with the purchase of the coloring solutions and also the purchase of color protection shampoos, or visits for touch-ups. If keeping your hair color is important, then go forth with coloring. Otherwise, keep it natural and just well-cut. Women love the distinguished look. Think George Clooney!

"Then you will look and be radiant, your heart will throb and swell with joy; the wealth on the seas will be brought to you, to you the riches of the nations will come."
Isaiah 60:5

Chapter 24

Oh, What Beautiful Hands You Have!

This is one of the nicest compliments I believe a woman or man can receive. You must take care of these two important friends. The skin on hands is thin and therefore fragile. If hands look old & frail, they can really age you. Hands are oh, so visible and you deserve yours to look lovely and youthful.

We need to take care of our hands. They do the work of the Lord!
You tell me that you moisturize, moisturize, moisturize. I have a better idea . . . Lets REJUVENATE our hands!
We spend so much time and money taking care of our face but we don't take time for our hands. It's easy: whatever you apply to your face, apply to your hands.

- For thin skin on the hands and wrinkles a retinol product works well. Hands will begin to look firmer & fuller
- A hand scrub exfoliates old skin cells & makes skin look youthful
- Glycolic acid speeds cell turnover and is great for hands!
- Always put SPF on your hands
- Again, anything you have left on your hands after you apply to your face, rub it in

Here's My Hand Regimen

Step 1: I love a good Glycolic Acid product. I have one that I use faithfully called Rejuvenate TR. When I apply it to my face, I bring it down to my neck, then apply it to my hands. Glycolic Acid will help diminish age spots or sun spots and promote cell turn-over and slough off dead skin cells for softer skin. Skin appears more hydrated and youthful glow returns.

Step 2: Ester-C (Not ascorbic acid) - I love Ester-C because it protects against sun damage and will also lessen the appearance of uneven skin pigmentation. Ester-C can increase skin's elasticity and skin becomes firmer and wrinkles fill in. Even if I'm using an SPF on my hands I will additionally apply Ester-C. I also dab on a little DMAE cream.

Step 3: While I'm applying my night serum or cream, I just get that extra cream left on my fingers & apply it to my hands.

Step 4: If your hands are really dry, find a product with hyaluronic acid. Hyaluronic acid acts like a sponge and increases the moisture content of the outer layer of the skin almost immediately. It is capable of retaining up to 6,000 times its weight in water! Your skin will instantly look hydrated.

Barbara's Hand Commandments

- Always apply sunscreen with SPF 30
- Hyaluronic acid is your best hydrator. Moisturizing hands will help them look younger because it plumps up the skin
- Glycolic acid will restore a youthful glow
- Vitamin C-ester increases collagen to thicken the skin
- Take Vitamin E? Break an extra softgel & apply to hands
- If you use a DMAE product, it will also firm your hand skin

I want your hands to look as good as your face. After all, people are ALWAYS looking at your hands.

I have been living in sunny southern California for over 30 years and I am really pleased that I do not have any age spots or sun spots on my hands! This is because I have been taking good care of my hands. It so easy, you don't have to buy a single extra product. Just apply what you're using on your face to your hands!

When you get all done, have some fun! Get some big colorful rings. Show off your gorgeous hands and be proud!

"I desire then that in every place the men should pray, lifting holy hands without anger or quarreling."
1 Timothy 2:8

Chapter 25

Younger, Sparkling Eyes

Youthful eyes are bright, clear and have a twinkle.
Older eyes can become dry, making them look dull.

Do your eyes feel like they have sand in them?
If the feeling is almost constant, that is called Dry Eye
Syndrome.

Dry Eye Syndrome is one of the most common complaints
heard by eye doctors. DES affects about 77 million people,
especially women, over the age of 40. More than 60% of
women suffer from dry eyes at a ratio of 9:1 over men.
If you have ever experienced dry eyes, you know how
miserable it feels. Here are the most effective natural
supplements to alleviate dry eyes.

Essential Fatty Acids – These are key. You want to include
omega-3 and omega-6. They can lower risk of developing dry
eyes by 68%! They can also reduce existing symptoms.

Zinc – This element is vital in the construction of a healthy
corneal surface. The highest concentration of zinc in the entire
body is in the cornea of the eye. So "Think Zinc" to nourish dry
eyes.

Magnesium & Vitamin E – Magnesium helps the body
produce a hormone called prostaglandine E-7, which is
necessary for tear production. Vitamin E aids in the proper
absorption of magnesium. Usually within 6 weeks, the tear film
is hydrated again.

Natural Progesterone – In a March 2007 study in Bologna,
Italy researchers determined that the eye's surface dryness
and inflammation were significantly related to the estrogen
peak occurring during the follicular phase.

Using natural progesterone can help keep estrogen in balance. Again, progesterone to the rescue!

For great tips on eye make-up go to Part II – Chapter 22. No dry eyes for us! We want eyes that sparkle!

"The eye is the lamp of the body. So, if your eye is healthy, your whole body will be full of light."
Matthew 6:22

Chapter 26

You're On Your Way!
Say Hello To The
Younger You

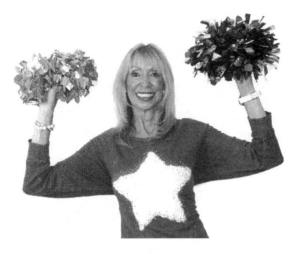

There!
Now you know what I know about feeling and looking younger.
You don't need to make any drastic changes. A few
well-chosen tweaks and you can be a Younger You. I promise.

Well, friends, this book had to come to an end eventually.
I found that I could just keep adding and adding.
I LOVE research, health, skin care, and all things that keep us
looking and feeling young.

I want us all to be the 90 year-olds who are zipping around
town looking & feeling fabulous.
The longer we live, the more God can use us and, I, for one,
want to feel as good as I can as I do His work.

By the way, a friend once said to me, "Barbara, if there was an after-life, you would definitely come back as an exclamation point."
Yes, I'm sure you notice. That's because I am so enthusiastic about my life which I devote to helping others. I hope you didn't mind!

I get lots of questions in a single day . . . by phone, fax, email, and on Facebook. I love them all. I am a researcher & teacher at heart.
Please don't hesitate to call me. My staff will track me down.
I'm here for you . . . the Younger You!

So, in order to continue sharing with you, I have a category on my Hope For Your Hormones blog called YOUNGER YOU.
I will keep it updated and you can leave your comments and tips and we can all move forward together!
P.S. there is some other great information about hormones on the blog and also some of my favorite recipes.

I'm going to miss "talking to you" thru this book, so please keep in touch!

Much Love,
Barbara Hoffman
Corona del Mar, CA 2013

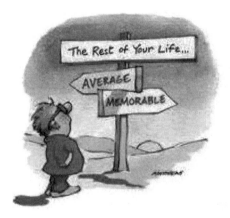

Barbara's Supplements Glossary

5-HTP – 5-HTP (5-hydroxytryptophan) is a metabolite of the amino acid tryptophan. Tryptophan is broken down by vitamins, enzymes, and other co-factors into 5-HTP, 5-HTP is then turned into serotonin. 5-HTP has been extensively researched for the treatment of depression & anxiety. 5-HTP's natural relief for depression & related problems, without the side effects of pharmaceutical alternatives.

EFAs – Essential Fatty Acids help the body produce hormones, lubricates eyes, helps regulate cholesterol, and is found to be effective for depression. EFAs contain anti-inflammatory compounds that relieve arthritis and autoimmune diseases. They can block tumor formation. The 3 types of EFAs are: Omega-3, Omega-6, & Omega-9.

DHEA – DHEA is made by the adrenal glands and is converted into male and female hormones. It can raise testosterone levels. Declining levels are believed to be associated with age-related diseases such as memory loss and heart disease. It can also help with depression, bone health, and "belly fat".

Folic Acid – Folic Acid is one of the most common vitamin deficiencies. It is water soluble, so daily consumption is necessary. Low folic acid levels have been associated with Alzheimer's disease. It is also great for depression and pre-menstrual syndrome.

L-Tyrosine – L-Tyrosine increases the rate at which the brain produces dopamine and norepinepherine (natural anti-depressants). It is essential for normal thyroid hormone production. Some prescription medications for depression work by boosting L-Tyrosine levels in the brain.

GABA – Gamma-aminobutyric acid (GABA) is an amino acid that is the second most prevalent neurotransmitter in the brain. GABA has an inhibiting effect, calming excited nerve impulses. Great for anxiety and also calm concentration.

Glutathione – Gluathione is one of the body's primary and most important antioxidants to help protect against free-radical damage.
It converts fat-soluble heavy metals and toxins into water-soluble waste, which can be excreted by the kidneys. Glutathione is essential for liver detoxification. It is found in virtually every cell in the body as well as in the fluid that surrounds the lens of the eye.

Milk Thistle – Milk Thistle is an anti-oxidant, anti-inflammatory herb containing bioflavonoids. The active agent of milk thistle is silymarin, which acts as a powerful antioxidant for the liver. It can stimulate growth of new liver cells. Cleanses the liver and enhances function.

SAM-e – SAM-e is made in the liver from the amino acid methionine. It can increase brain levels of dopamine and serotonin. Used widely in Europe. SAM-e has been found effective in treatment of depression.

Phosphatidylserine (PS) – PS is a phospholipid (fat) that helps support the brain and its function. PS helps relay messages between the cells of the brain and helps the brain retrieve messages. Levels of PS in the brain decrease with age. Studies show PS improves memory.

Vitamin D – Vitamin D is known as the 'sunshine vitamin" because the sun's ultraviolet rays act in the skin to produce vitamin D, which is then absorbed by the body. Many people over the age of 45 are found to be deficient in Vitamin D. It is essential for the maintenance of bone density. Without vitamin D, calcium cannot be utilized to build bones.

Melatonin – Melatonin is a hormone secreted by the pineal gland within the brain. When normal, it's levels peak at night and fall during the day, creating the body's sleep/wake cycle. The level of melatonin in the body decreases with age. Melatonin is best known for its role in promoting sleep. Other studies show that it may also slow the effects of aging. It plays an important roll in immune function by activating cancer-fighting cells.

Progesterone – In 1936, Japanese scientists used an extraction process and discovered dioscorea from the wild Mexican yam plant.
It was found that the chemical configuration was almost identical to the progesterone excreted by the female ovaries. The United States Pharmacopoeia then standardized this to the form we know today as natural progesterone or USP progesterone.
Progesterone levels decline to almost zero as a woman approaches or enters menopause. Progesterone is the natural balance to estrogen in the body and is also necessary for the body's optimum use of the good estrogen that it makes.

Rhodiola – Rhodiola Rosea is a powerful adaptogenic herb known for its beneficial effects on energy production and reduction of fatigue. Rhodiola is great for increasing your energy levels and enhancing your mental and physical performance. Adaptogens like Rhodiola actually support proper adrenal function and help the adrenal glands produce cortisol in natural patterns.

Barbara's Make-up Glossary

These are the Younger You brand.
You could look for similar products.

Concealer

Duo- Corrector Concealer – Neutralize dark circles with a duo-shaded concealer. No matter what color skin you have (from very pale to dark brown) concealer should be one or two shades lighter than your skin. Our Duo Concealer provides the perfect combo of yellow tones that help lighten darkness under the eyes.

Eye Shadow
Indelible Crème Eye Shadow

Unbelievably Fabulous! These sophisticated, highly-pigmented crème shadows glide on smooth & dry instantly for a beautiful, fixed finish. Waterproof, crease proof and long wearing. These are my favorites for you! Hand selected from over 30 products.

Bare Necessity – Beautiful matte, "ballet" pink
Spun Silk – Golden beige, slight shimmer
Bronze Frost – Shimmery Cappuccino brown
Sweet Dreams – Shimmery, girly pink
Ever After – Charming soft, silvery purple
Moon Walk – Rich gray-brown, slight shimmer

Eye Liner
Ultimate Eye Liner Pencils

Take your eyes to the max! Vitamin enriched, super smooth formula. Long lasting and waterproof, these pencils glide on and stay on all day without smearing.

Gravity – A gray-black-blue combination
Libido – A lush, royal purple, but fine for everyday
Meteor – Charcoal black with gold flecks

Slim Eye Pencils

For a more understated look. These "slims" line your eyes with ease and glide on effortlessly for a beautiful, precise line.

156

Cocoa Bronze – A warm, nutmeg brown
Midnight – A dark & stormy blue with gray undertones

Lashes

If your lashes are thin, mascara is your best beauty secret! There is no need for thin lashes in this age of cosmetics. One or two coats of mascara will make your eyes look large and brighter. These products will give you gorgeous lashes at affordable prices.

Mascara with Keratin

A vitamin-enrich application for your lashes. Flake-free, long wearing, smudge-proof. Not too thick, so no clumping.
Intense Black & Rich Brown

Ultimate Volume Mascara

Turn up the volume! Provides plush, thick lashes with lash extending fibers. Flake-free, long wearing, smudge proof.
Intense Black & Rich Brown

Tinted Moisturizers

Hydrating, oil-free formula. Restores skin's essential moisture and provides natural sheer coverage. SPF 15, Vitamin A, C, and E help protect the skin from free radicals and other harmful environmental toxins. Hyaluronic Acid hydrates the skin. Vitamin B5 and Allantoin soothe irritation and help keep skin clear. For all skin types! If desired, they can be mixed with your current foundation for heavier, dewy coverage.

Touch of Sand (Light) – Fair Ivory skin tones
Touch of Sun (Medium) – Beige skin tones
Touch of Radiance (Olive) – Olive Skin Tones
Touch of Tan (Dark) – Dark Skin Tones or when you have a tan

Cheeks
Crème Blush
Super soft & creamy formula. Glides on effortlessly for a creamy glow. Water resistant formulas stay on all day.

Lullaby – Beautiful, pinkish-apricot
Flaunt – Rich pink, coral undertones
Showoff – Neutral sun-kissed bronzer

Collage Powders
These silky powders offer the best variety of shades that blend together for bronzing, highlighting, and evening out skin tones. Collage Powders diffuse light for a soft and youthful glow!

Matisse – A beautiful variety of rosy shades and pigments that blend to give a soft and youthful pink glow
Soliel – Combines shades of bronze to create the perfect California, sun-kissed look
Soft Glow – Don't want color? This reflective powder will give you a fresh, dewy look. Use to highlight and add a finished, polished look to your makeup or use alone.

Lips
Liquid Lips
Our favorite lip stain / lipstick / gloss. Soaks your lips in high shine for totally glam looking lips. Enriched with Vitamin E, this gloss leaves lips soft and luscious. Non-sticky, glossy, weightless formula stays shiny and fresh! It will stay on for 6 plus hours!

Red Carpet – Best red I have found! Suits anyone age 15 to 115.
Cranberry –A shimmery vibrant cranberry. Great for day and night.
Beloved – Pinkish nude color, makes lips look kissably sweet.
Nude Plum – Don't want pink? Mauvey-nude shade with shimmer.

Lip Enhancer

Formulated to increase the size of the lips. Contains the vaso dilator Niacin, a vitamin B derivative that increases blood flow and improves circulation to the lips. The niacin provides instant lip plumping that works in 1-2 minutes and lasts for hours.
It also contains peptides, which are amino acids that, with continued use, will stimulate the production of collagen and hyaluronic acid for long term lip plumping.

Clear – Great finishing gloss to wear over lipstick, lip stain or alone.
Crystal Rose – Shimmery, dusty red

"You are altogether beautiful, my darling,
and there is no blemish in you."
Song of Solomon 4:7

Need Help with Weight?

Barbara's *Eat Yourself Slender* has the answers for YOU!

No More:
- ✓ **Deprivation**
- ✓ **Counting calories**
- ✓ **Starving Yourself**
- ✓ **Yo-Yo dieting**

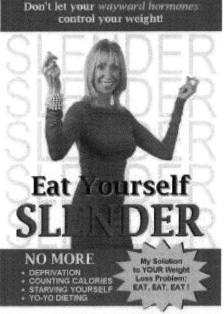

Kindle Version Available on Amazon
Or Get Your Copy at www.bhnformulas.com
Or By Calling 877-880-0170

Made in the USA
Lexington, KY
18 June 2016